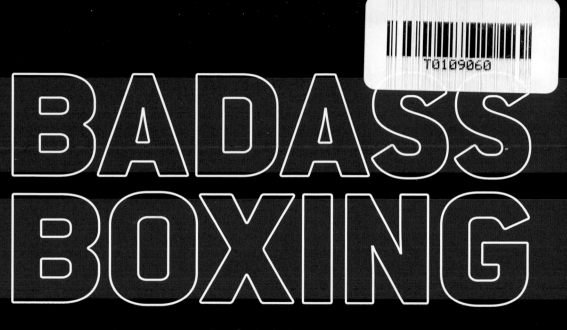

BADASS BOXING

• WORKOUTS •

BADASS
BOXING
· WORKOUTS ·

A HARD-HITTING PROGRAM TO SMASH STRESS, HAVE FUN & GET IN THE BEST SHAPE OF YOUR LIFE

JENNIFER DUGWEN CHIENG

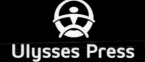

Ulysses Press

Published in the United States by:
Ulysses Press
P.O. Box 3440
Berkeley, CA 94703
www.ulyssespress.com

ISBN: 978-1-61243-875-7

Library of Congress Control Number: 2018959347

Printed in Korea by Artin Printing Company through Four Colour Print Group
10 9 8 7 6 5 4 3 2 1

Acquisitions: Bridget Thoreson
Managing editor: Claire Chun
Project editor: Claire Sielaff
Editor: Shayna Keyles
Proofreader: Renee Rutledge
Indexer: Sayre Van Young
Front cover design: Raquel Castro
Interior design and layout: what!design @ whatweb.com
Photographs: © Joshua Brandenburg
Models: Jennifer Dugwen Chieng, Bridget Grace, Raquel Harris, Henry Lee

Distributed by Publishers Group West

Please Note: This book has been written and published strictly for informational purposes, and in no way should be used as a substitute for consultation with health care professionals. You should not consider educational material herein to be the practice of medicine or to replace consultation with a physician or other medical practitioner. The author and publisher are providing you with information in this work so that you can have the knowledge and can choose, at your own risk, to act on that knowledge. The author and publisher also urge all readers to be aware of their health status and to consult health care professionals before beginning any health program. This book is independently authored and published and no sponsorship or endorsement of this book by, and no affiliation with, any trademarked brands or other products mentioned or pictured within is claimed or suggested. All trademarks that appear in this book belong to their respective owners and are used here for informational purposes only. The author and publisher encourage readers to patronize the quality brands and other products mentioned and pictured in this book.

CONTENTS

INTRODUCTION

I want to commend you for taking initiative toward a healthy and active lifestyle. I am excited to help guide and challenge you in your journey to reach your fitness goals by developing your boxing skill set.

My intention for this book is twofold. First, I hope that undertaking the challenge to learn a new skill set gives you a sense of empowerment, as it did for me when I first started boxing years ago. Embracing new challenges is key to revealing capabilities and unfolding your potential, whether you are a competitive athlete or a hobbyist. Second, this book aims to fill in the intricate details of boxing technique, and concepts, which are simple in theory, yet often prove to be challenging in execution. Throwing a punch, for example, is the simple concept of connecting a maximum amount of generated force to a perceived target. The real challenge falls with your ability to coordinate and control your movement. Developing this ability requires a great amount of time and patience, a diligent effort, and of course, the application of proper body mechanics to ensure effective and efficient execution. Moreover, understanding how to control your movement using proper form and weight distribution helps prevent injury.

As a former Olympic boxer and current mixed martial artist, it took me years to develop my skill set. I continue to work on my craft as a life-long learner of martial arts. That's the beauty of martial arts—learning does not stop with your achievements; you can only improve. With this in mind, let's embark on this journey together!

USING THIS BOOK

This book will provide detailed instructions on boxing techniques that can be incorporated into a fitness regimen. It starts by familiarizing you with a list of boxing terminology. We will examine techniques, including basic punches such as the jab, cross, hook, and uppercut, and we will build upon each of these punches to create multiple sequences or combinations utilizing efficient movement. You will also learn how to generate power and speed in your punches. It is important for you to understand the proper body mechanics that maximize the impact absorbed by the target from any given punch.

The book will also emphasize detail in footwork, as footwork is the foundation of effective offense and defense. Additionally, developing a solid foundation in footwork is fundamental to learning how to connect your punches with a moving target at a high rate. Although this book assumes a stationary target for beginner learning purposes, the exercises within apply to both moving and stationary targets alike. Techniques in the footwork section include movement and striking along various planes of motion (frontal, sagittal, transverse), as well as how to pivot, advance, retreat, and understand weight distribution and balance. In terms of defensive techniques, the book will examine basic methods to avoid punches through slips, dips, catch and throw, parries, circles, and pivots. You'll learn how to incorporate these techniques when shadowboxing to further develop muscle memory, rhythm, and coordination.

Following the introduction of punches and footwork, you will be guided through several exercises designed to gradually develop the muscle memory necessary for each technique. As we move into the shadowboxing portion of the book, you will gain an understanding of the essential role it plays in helping develop skill areas such as effective punching technique, generating power through speed, muscular endurance, and balance and stability. The exercises in the later sections include punch combinations, footwork, defensive technique, and other plyometric exercises designed to address development in each of these skill areas.

Taking into consideration that this might be your first attempt at boxing, we will also address adjustments to correct common mistakes that occur, such as leaning too far forward, leaning too far backward, or overextending when throwing punches. As you continue to develop your boxing competency, in addition to improved coordination and efficient movement, you will naturally begin to increase the intensity of these exercises, which is important for a higher output of work.

As this book aims to establish a strong foundation for beginners, we will examine boxing fundamentals assuming a stationary target. Therefore, this book will exclude the following advanced concepts that require execution on a moving target:

1. Managing time and distance

2. Offensive and defensive strategies based on technical style of a moving target

3. Advanced offensive and defensive strategies based on physical attributes of a moving target

4. Controlling distance and influencing the direction of a moving target

5. Feints

6. Advanced defensive and offensive technique

7. Advanced footwork and ring control

8. Advanced counterpunching technique

In this chapter, we define specific phrases and words to help familiarize you with boxing terminology.

Boxing stance: Your boxing stance is your neutral and ready position. There are two types of boxing stances: orthodox and southpaw. Orthodox stance is favored by right-handed boxers, while southpaw stance is favored by left-handed boxers.

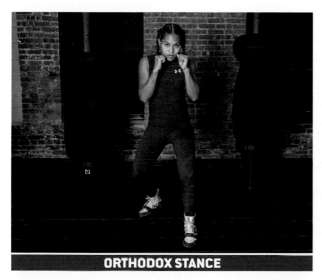

ORTHODOX STANCE

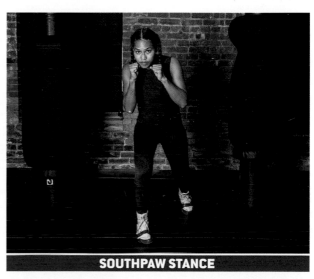

SOUTHPAW STANCE

For an *orthodox stance*, start with your feet shoulder-width apart and take one step back with your right foot. The toes of your right foot (rear foot) should be pointed at a 45-degree angle while the toes of your left foot (lead foot) should be pointed straight forward. Your knees should be slightly bent. Slightly curve your back by rounding your shoulders. Tuck in your chin and your elbows, keeping minimal space between the arms and rib cage. Making a relaxed fist with both hands, bring your left fist close to the left side of your chin and your right fist close to the right side of your chin.

For a *southpaw stance*, start with your feet shoulder-width apart and take one step back with your left foot. The toes of your left foot (rear foot) should be pointed at a 45-degree angle while the toes of your right foot (lead foot) should be pointed straight forward. Your knees should be slightly bent. Slightly curve your back by rounding your shoulders. Tuck in your chin and your elbows, keeping minimal space between the arms and rib cage. Making a relaxed fist with both hands, bring your left fist close to the left side of your chin and your right fist close to the right side of your chin.

While most of the boxing exercises in this book are demonstrated in the orthodox stance, I use the term "neutral stance" or "boxing stance" in the instructions to indicate the ready position. Chapters 4 and 5 do offer drill variations for those who prefer using the southpaw stance.

Target: The target is a set point to connect your punches to. You may set specific points on a physical target, such as a boxing heavy bag or boxing mitts. If you do not have access to a boxing heavy bag, you may set specific points on a perceived target in the air (see Shadowboxing on page 13). Target areas include:

- Frontal plane: Anterior (front) of target's face and body
- Left sagittal plane: Left lateral aspect (side) of target's face and body
- Right sagittal plane: Right lateral aspect (side) of target's face and body
- Bottom transverse plane: Bottom of target's face

Extension: Extension increases the inner angle of a joint. Throwing a punch requires muscle extension around the elbow joint to enable your turned closed fist to travel in a forward direction from its starting position at your chin toward the desired target. Every punch requires a certain degree of muscle extension to connect to a desired target.

Flexion: Flexion decreases the inner angle of a joint. Retracting a punch requires muscle flexion around the elbow joint to enable your turned closed fist to reset, or travel back, from the target to its starting position at your chin.

Retraction: Retraction is active flexion on an extended punch. In other words, retraction is withdrawing your turned closed fist back to your chin after connecting to the desired target through extension. In boxing, this is best known through the expression "keep your hands up."

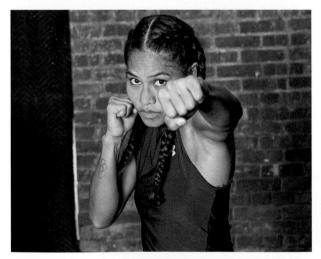 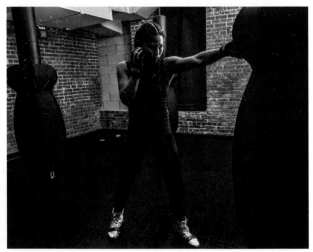

Jab: Your jab is thrown by your lead hand (the hand that is closest to the target). If you are in orthodox stance, your jab will be thrown by your left hand. If you are in southpaw stance, your jab will be thrown by your right hand. Keep your elbows tucked in close to your body and ensure that you connect with your knuckles by rotating your wrist so that your thumb is facing down. Aim to strike the frontal plane of your target with your jab. To throw an up-jab, lower your lead forearm so your fist is level with your naval. Lock your elbow at an angle slightly wider than 90 degrees.

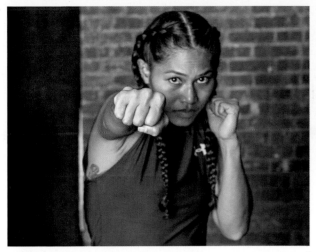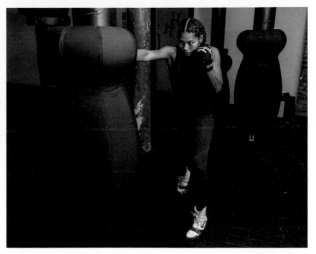

Cross: Your cross is the punch thrown by the rear hand (the hand that is closest to your face). If you are in orthodox stance, your cross will be thrown by your right hand, while taking on a southpaw stance will require the use of your left hand to deliver the punch. Keep your elbows tucked in close to your body and connect with your knuckles by rotating your wrist so that your thumb is facing down. Aim to strike the frontal plane of your target with your cross.

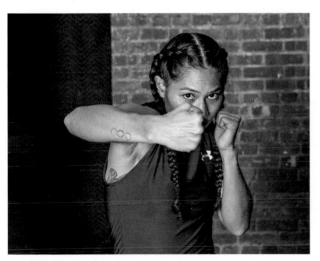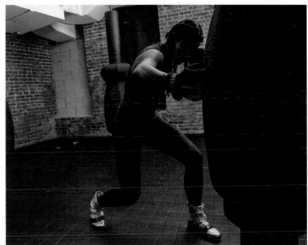

Right hook: Execute the right hook by lifting your right elbow until it is parallel to your shoulder. Keep an approximately 90-degree bend in your elbow. Hold your arm in this position as you rotate around the waist while slightly pivoting on the toes of your rear foot to ease through the rotation. With a closed fist and thumb facing up, ensure you are striking the left sagittal plane of your target with your knuckles.

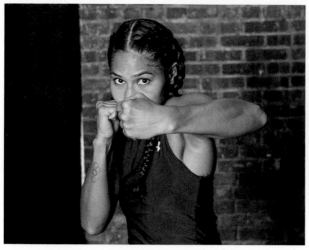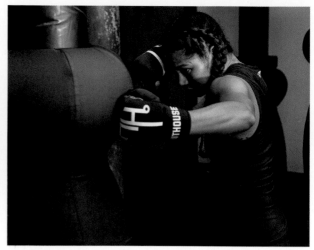

Left hook: Execute the left hook by lifting your left elbow until it is parallel to your shoulder. Keep an approximately 90-degree bend in your elbow. Hold your arm in this position as you rotate around the waist while slightly pivoting on the toes of your lead foot to ease through the rotation. With a closed fist and thumb facing up, ensure you are striking the right sagittal plane of your target with your knuckles.

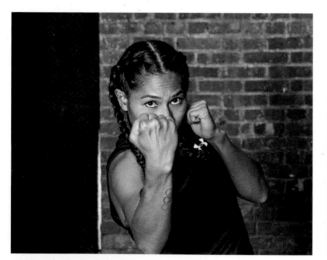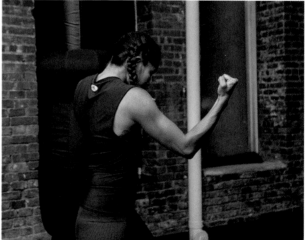

Right uppercut: The right uppercut is executed by striking the bottom transverse plane of your target. From your boxing stance, lower your right forearm until the angle of your elbow is between 30 and 90 degrees. Rotate around your waist and pivot slightly on the ball of your rear foot as you throw the punch upward and outward to strike your target with the knuckles of your fist.

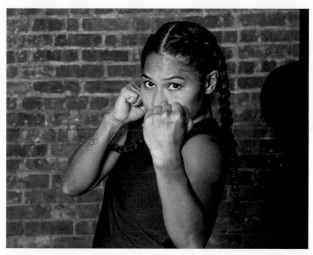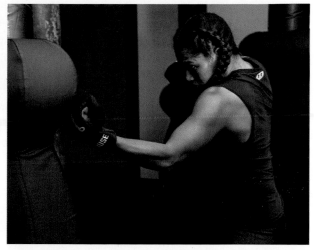

Left uppercut: The left uppercut is executed by striking the bottom transverse plane of your target. From your boxing stance, lower your left forearm until the angle of your elbow is between 30 and 90 degrees. Rotate around your waist and pivot slightly on the ball of your rear foot as you throw the punch upward and outward to strike your target with the knuckles of your fist.

Shadowboxing: Shadowboxing is the active effort to improve accuracy and effective execution of technique by practicing on a perceived target (as opposed to a physical target, such as a heavy bag or opponent). You train to use correct form and body mechanics despite changing variables in speed, timing, resistance, etc. See page 81 for more details.

Pivot: The pivot is a rotating motion on the balls of your feet along the transverse plane. This book will address two types of pivoting actions: pivoting to change direction, and pivoting to add reach.

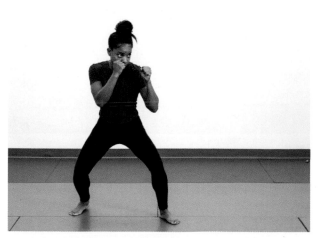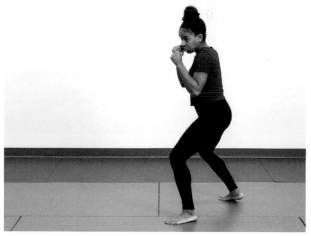

To pivot and change the direction that you are facing, push your rear foot into the floor to generate force in a forward motion. Redirect this force by rotating on the ball of your lead foot so that your entire body makes a 90-degree change in the angle you are currently facing.

You can also *pivot to add reach to punches*. Notice that in your boxing stance, your rear hand is farther away from the target than your lead hand. To compensate for the minor shortage of reach, slightly pivot on the ball of the rear foot so your toes change from pointing at a 45-degree angle to pointing directly forward at your target. This rotating motion when throwing a punch allows your hips and shoulders to shift a few degrees forward, subsequently adding reach to your rear hand.

Step off: Starting in your boxing stance, a step off occurs when one foot steps away from point A to point B and then back to point A while the other foot remains in its original position throughout. As this motion occurs, your head and body will no longer be directly in the center line of your target. Place your body weight on the foot stepping off.

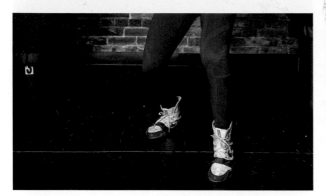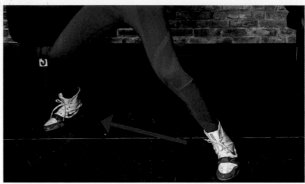

To *step off to the right*, the right foot moves from point A to point B and then back to point A. The left foot remains in its original position. To ensure you are distributing your body weight on the right foot, lift your left foot up slightly. If you can do so then you are distributing your weight correctly.

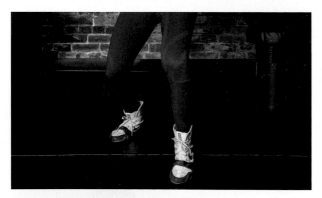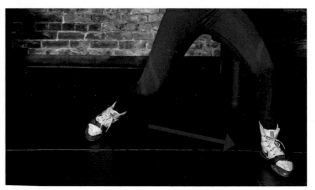

To *step off to the left*, the left foot moves from point A to point B and then back to point A. The right foot remains in its original position. To ensure you are distributing your body weight on the left foot, lift your right foot up slightly. If you can do so then you are distributing your weight correctly.

Step: A step occurs when both feet move from point A to point B, taking your entire body off your target's center line. This means your head and body will not be directly in line with your target. You are either stepping to the right or left to shift your body and head away from the target's center line. Take both feet with you so that your entire body is off the center line.

Center line: The center line is the perceived line that runs directly down the middle of your forward-facing target, splitting it into two equal halves. When standing in your boxing stance, the toes of your lead foot should be placed on the center line and point directly toward your forward-facing target.

Bob and weave: Bobbing and weaving are actions in which your head moves from side to side and up and down, away from the center line. Bobbing occurs when you rotate around the waist while alternating your shoulders in a slight forward slipping motion. Weaving occurs when you simultaneously rotate around the waist while lowering then raising your level through flexion and extension of the knees in such a way that the side-to-side movement of your head appears to make the shape of a "U." (See more about changing level on page 40; see the Weave Side to Side exercise on page 44.)

Slip: To slip a straight punch, you must take your head off the center line of attack by bending laterally around the waist.

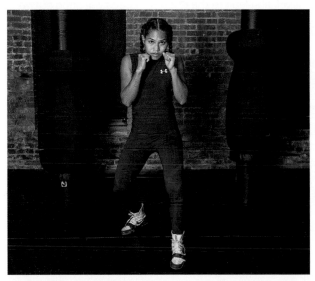 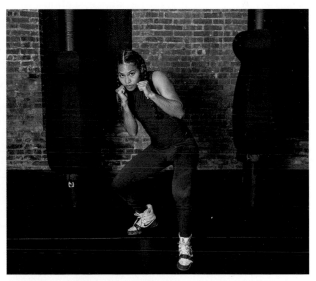

To *slip right*, start from your boxing stance, slightly lower your level, and lean to the right. Your knees bend outward and away from each other as you change your level. Your head and upper body shift away from the center line as you bend at the waist to lean to the right.

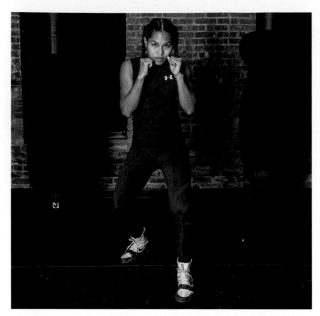
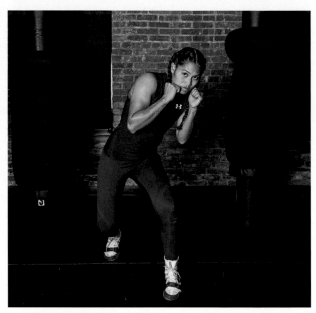

To *slip left*, start from your boxing stance, slightly lower your level, and lean to the left. Your knees will bend outward and away from each other as you change your level. Your head and upper body will shift away from the center line as you bend at the waist to lean to the left.

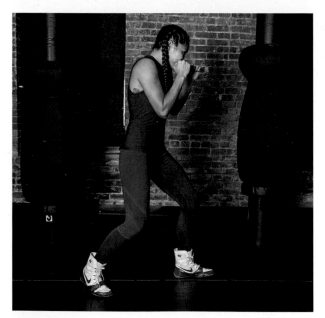
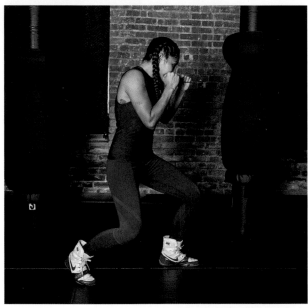

Dip: From your boxing stance, quickly lower your level by bending your knees to drop down then catching your weight once you've reached a lowered squat position. Extend your knees to bring yourself back into your initial starting position.

Shuffle: Shuffling your feet involves moving or shifting your body from one point to another by quickly sliding your feet along the floor.

Pendulum step: When in a staggered stance, the rear foot moves toward the lead foot. As the lead foot lifts and moves forward, the rear foot replaces the lead foot's former position. Similar mechanics apply when going forward, backward, and side to side. The key to this movement is maintaining your weight directly over your center of gravity.

Bounce: Bouncing, or "staying light on your feet," is an efficient method used to quickly shift movement in any direction, as speed is generated by motion—the conversion of potential energy to kinetic energy. This speed is simply redirected when needed. The ability to quickly shift movement in any direction is possible even without the bounce (see Chapter 2: Footwork).

From your boxing stance, bounce up and down on the balls of your feet. At this point your body weight is evenly distributed between your lead and rear feet. Shift your body weight back and forth between your lead and rear feet. Keep alternating your body weight between the lead foot and the rear foot as you bounce.

Guard: Defense technique that provides protection against punches to the head and body. In your boxing stance, your hands should be positioned by your chin to protect against punches to the head while your elbows should be positioned by your waist to protect against punches to the body.

FOOTWORK

Developing a solid foundation in footwork is fundamental to connecting your punches to a moving target. In Chapter 1 we reviewed that your target could take a physical shape, such as a boxing heavy bag or boxing mitts, or it could be perceived, such as in shadowboxing. For perceived targets, you must still utilize correct form and body mechanics to develop the correct muscle memory required to effectively execute technique. In this chapter, we will assume a stationary target for learning purposes, but keep in mind that the exercises examined apply to both moving and stationary targets. Let's begin by incorporating terminology from the previous chapter into specific movements, starting with fundamentals in footwork.

Movement occurs along various planes of motion: the frontal plane, the sagittal plane, and the transverse plane.

Movement along the frontal plane is left to right (or side to side). Example: Standing with your feet parallel and face forward, take a step to the left and then to the right.

Movement along the sagittal plane is forward and backward. Example: Standing with your feet parallel and face forward, take a step forward and then backward.

Movement along the transverse plane is rotating. Example: Standing with your feet parallel and face forward, rotate around the waist to the left and then to the right.

To determine which foot takes the initial step from your boxing stance, you must first decide on the direction you wish to move. Generally, the foot closest to the direction you are moving will take the initial step, as it has the shortest distance to travel to reach the desired destination. The foot that takes this initial step is called the primary foot. The secondary foot follows and generates the "push" force required to drive the primary foot in the desired direction.

- Moving forward (advancing) along the sagittal plane: Your lead (primary) foot steps forward first and is followed by a step with the rear (secondary) foot.

- Moving backward (retreating) along the sagittal plane: Your rear (primary) foot steps backward first and is followed by a step with the lead (secondary) foot.

- Moving left along the frontal plane: Your left (primary) foot steps toward the left first and is followed by a step with the right (secondary) foot.

- Moving right along the frontal plane: Your right (primary) foot steps toward the right first and is followed by a step with the left (secondary) foot.

FORWARD, BACKWARD, LEFT, RIGHT

Starting in your boxing stance, take the following steps. Remember to take your first step with your primary foot and generate the "push" force with the secondary foot.

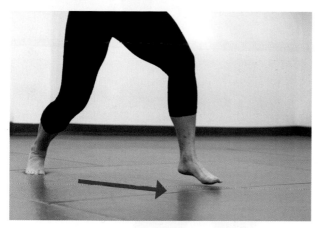 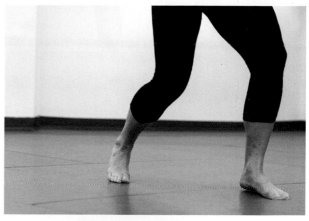

1. Advance. Your primary is your lead foot and your secondary is your rear foot.

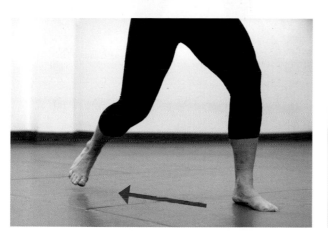 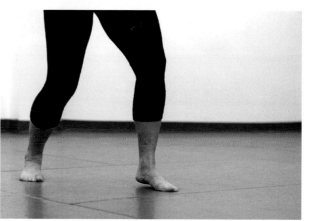

2. Retreat. Your primary is your rear foot and your secondary is your lead foot.

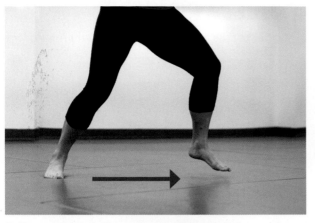 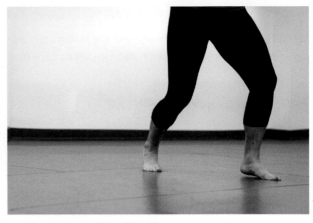

3. Step to the left. Your primary is your left foot and your secondary is your right foot.

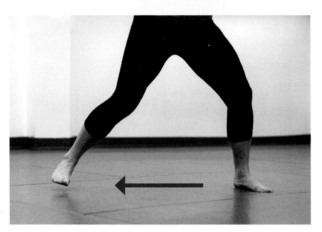 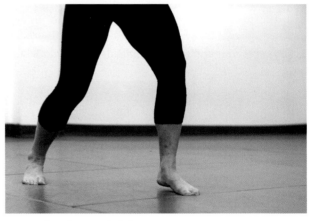

4. Step to the right. Your primary is your right foot and your secondary is your left foot.

Repeat this exercise until you can maintain a rhythm with this movement.

Note: When performing this exercise, start slowly and gradually increase your speed. Notice that pushing off your secondary foot increases your speed in the desired direction by converting potential energy into kinetic energy or, in other words, generating a propelling force behind the primary foot. After several repetitions, start to incorporate punches; add a jab, cross, and hook after each step.

UPPERCUTS MOVING FORWARD

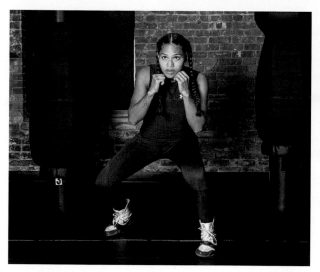 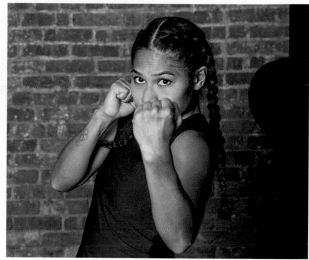

1. Starting in your boxing stance, take a step forward with your lead foot and begin to lower your level by bending your knees and weaving in the same direction as the lead foot.

2. As your knees begin to extend during the upward motion of the weave, throw an uppercut with your lead hand. Additionally, during the upward motion of the weave, take a step forward with your rear foot, resetting your boxing stance. At this point, your feet should be about shoulder-width apart.

3. Retract your lead hand to protect your chin.

4. Next, weave and take a lateral step with your rear foot.

5. As your knees begin to extend during the upward motion of the weave, throw an uppercut with your rear hand. During the upward motion of the weave, your lead foot takes a lateral step toward your rear foot, resetting your boxing stance. Your feet should be about shoulder-width apart.

6. Retract your rear hand back to protect your chin.

Important note: When following your lead foot, the rear foot takes a forward and diagonal step. Next, the rear foot takes a lateral step, followed by a lateral step of the lead foot in the same direction, which avoids bringing both feet parallel to each other.

UPPERCUTS MOVING BACKWARD

1. Starting in your boxing stance, take a step backward with your rear foot as you begin to lower your level by flexing your knees and weaving in the same direction as the rear foot.

2. As your knees begin to extend during the upward motion of the weave, throw an uppercut with your rear hand. During the upward motion of the weave, take a step backward with your lead foot to return to your boxing stance. At this point, the distance between your feet should be about shoulder-width apart.

3. Retract your rear hand to protect your chin.

4. Take a lateral step as you weave in the same direction as your lead foot.

5. As your knees begin to extend during the upward motion of the weave, throw an uppercut with your lead hand. During the upward motion of the weave, step your rear foot laterally, following the lead foot, to reset you into your boxing stance.

6. Retract your lead hand back to protect your chin.

Important note: When following your rear foot, the lead foot takes a backward and diagonal step. Next, the lead foot takes a lateral step followed by a lateral step of the rear foot in the same direction, which avoids bringing both feet parallel to each other.

JAB AND CROSS MOVING SIDE TO SIDE

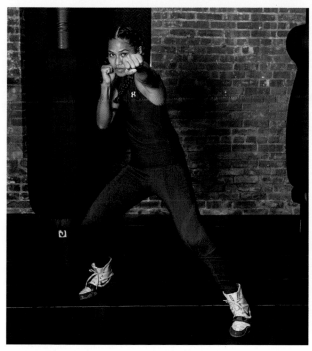 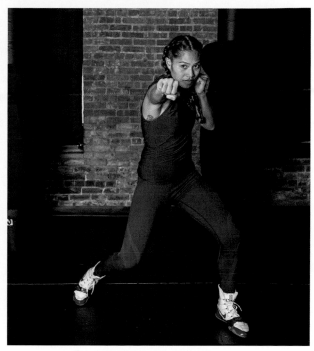

1. Starting in your boxing stance, take a lateral step in the direction of rear foot. Push off your lead foot, keeping it in starting position.

2. As you step off, extend your jab. Retract your jab as you push off your rear foot to step back to your starting position.

3. Step off in the lateral direction of your lead foot. Push off your rear foot, keeping it in starting position.

4. As you step off, extend your cross. Retract your cross as you push off your lead foot to step back to your starting position.

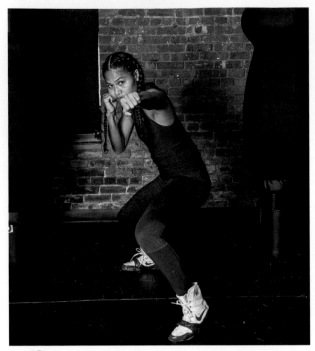 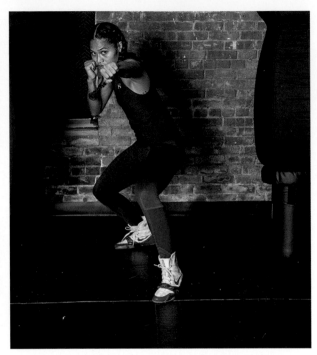

1. Starting in your boxing stance, step forward in the direction of your lead foot, keeping your rear foot in its starting position. As you begin to close distance with your desired target, extend your jab while slightly lowering your level.

2. Retract your jab as you push off your lead foot to step back to starting position. Bring your level back to starting position.

3. Step off in the direction of your rear foot, keeping your lead foot in its starting position. As you step off, extend your jab while slightly lowering your level.

4. Retract your jab as you push off your rear foot to step back to starting position. Bring your level back to starting position.

Note: For extra practice, combine this exercise with Jab and Cross Moving Side to Side (page 23).

JAB AND REAR UPPERCUT WITH REAR STEP OFF

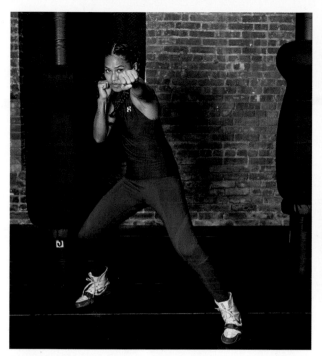 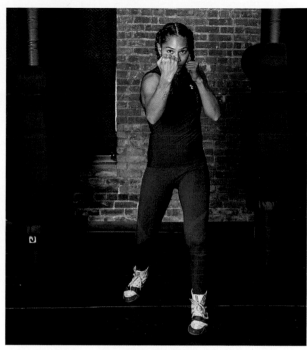

1. Starting in your boxing stance, take a step laterally in the direction of your rear foot. Keep your lead foot in its original position. As you step off, extend your jab.

2. Retract your jab as you push off your rear foot to return it back to its starting position.

3. As you push off your rear foot, throw a rear uppercut that connects with its target at the same time as your rear foot returns to its original position.

CROSS AND LEAD HOOK WITH LEAD STEP OFF

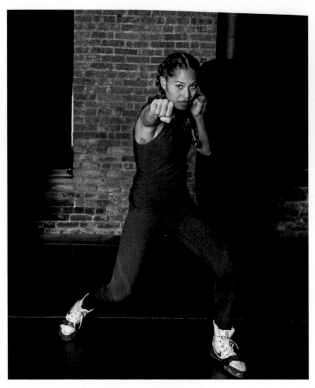 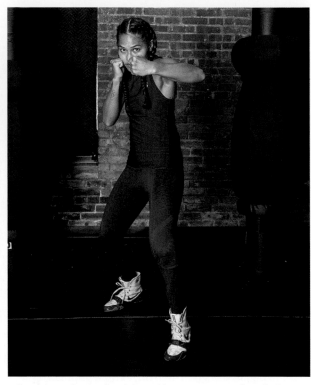

1. Starting in your boxing stance, take a step laterally in the direction of your lead foot. Keep your rear foot in its original position. As you step off, extend your cross.

2. Retract your cross as you push off your lead foot to return it back to its starting position.

3. As you push off your lead foot, throw a lead hook that connects with its target at the same time your lead foot returns to its original starting position.

Note: For extra practice, combine this move with Jab and Rear Uppercut with Rear Step Off (page 25).

PENDULUM STEP—FORWARD AND BACKWARD (ORTHODOX)

The aim of this exercise is to keep your entire body weight over a designated point, a perceived "X," by leaning on the foot that stands on the designated center point.

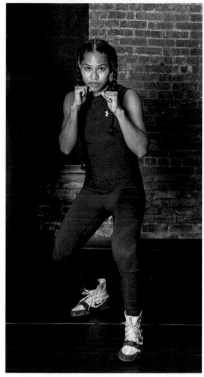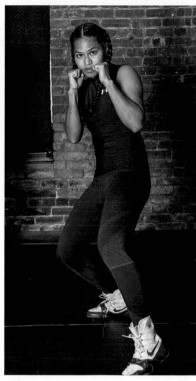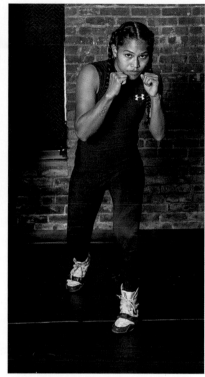

1. Start with your left (lead) foot on the perceived "X." Lean your weight directly over the left foot.

2. Keeping your weight over the "X," shuffle your feet to switch out your left foot with your right foot. Shift your weight to be directly over the right foot by leaning backward.

3. Return to your boxing stance by shuffling your feet so the left foot moves back over the perceived "X." Simultaneously shift your weight forward. Step the right foot back into its initial position.

Repeat this forward and backward movement along the sagittal plane, alternating the left and right foot on the "X" while shifting your weight over each respective foot, for 1 minute.

PENDULUM STEP—SIDE TO SIDE (ORTHODOX)

The aim of this exercise is to keep your entire body weight over a designated point, a perceived "X," by leaning on the foot that stands on the designated center point.

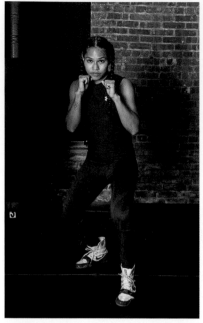 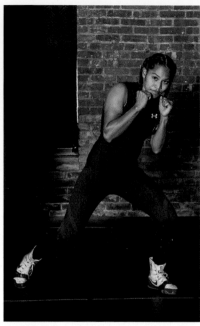 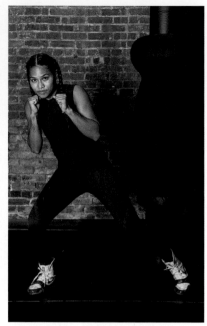

1. Start with your left (lead) foot on the perceived "X." Bring your feet parallel by stepping the rear foot forward, and lean your weight over the left foot.

2. Keeping your weight over the "X," shuffle your feet to switch out the left foot with your right foot. Lean to the right to shift your weight over your right foot.

3. Shuffle your feet to place the left foot onto the perceived "X," simultaneously leaning to the left and shifting your weight over your left foot.

Repeat this side-to-side movement along the frontal plane, alternating the left and right foot on the "X" while shifting your weight over each respective foot, for 1 minute.

PENDULUM STEP—FORWARD AND BACKWARD (SOUTHPAW)

The aim of this exercise is to keep your entire body weight over a designated point, a perceived "X," by leaning on the foot that stands on the designated center point.

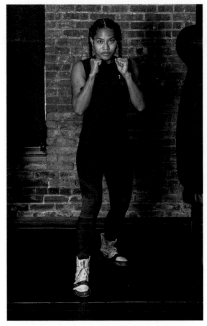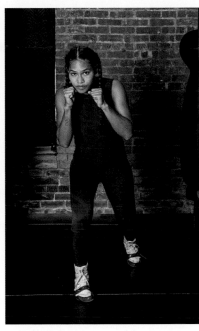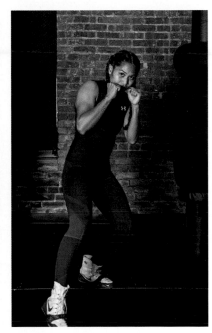

1. Start with your right (lead) foot on the perceived "X." Lean your weight over the right foot.

2. Keeping your weight over the "X," shuffle your feet to switch out your right foot with your left foot. Shift your weight to be directly over to the left foot by leaning backward.

3. Return to your boxing stance by shuffling your feet so the right foot moves back over the perceived "X." Simultaneously shift your weight forward. Step the left foot back into its initial position.

Repeat this forward and backward movement along the sagittal plane, alternating the right and left foot on the "X" while shifting your weight over each respective foot, for 1 minute.

PENDULUM STEP—SIDE TO SIDE (SOUTHPAW)

The aim of this exercise is to keep your entire body weight over a designated point, a perceived "X," by leaning on the foot that stands on the designated center point.

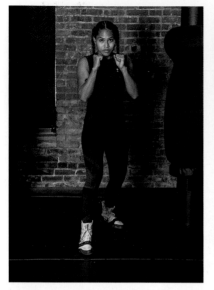 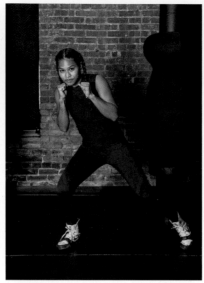 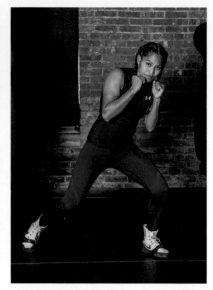

1. Start with your right (lead) foot on the perceived "X." Bring your feet parallel by stepping your rear foot forward, and lean your weight over the right foot.

2. Keeping your weight over the "X," shuffle your feet to switch out the right foot with your left foot. Lean to the left to shift your weight over your left foot.

3. Shuffle your feet to place the right foot back on the perceived "X," simultaneously leaning to the right and shifting your weight over your right foot.

Repeat this side-to-side movement along the frontal plane, alternating the right and left foot on the "X" while shifting your weight over each respective foot, for 1 minute.

PIVOT

Pivoting involves movement along the transverse plane. This movement is especially useful when trying to redirect an opposing force through changes in the direction you are facing.

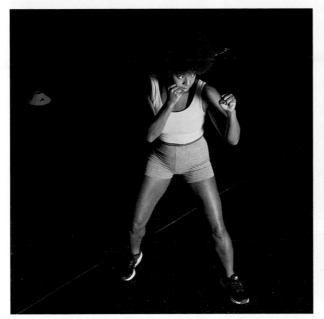
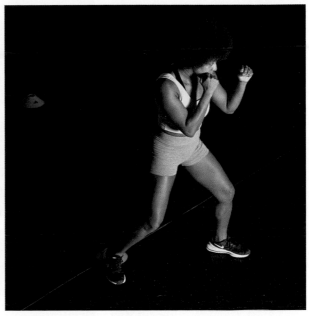

1. Push off your lead foot to generate momentum in your rear foot as you rotate 90 degrees on the ball of your rear foot.

2. Next, push off your rear foot to generate momentum in your lead foot as you rotate 90 degrees on the ball of your lead foot. Both the degree and direction of your pivot may vary depending on your preference and on the situation.

3. Practice pivoting in both directions as well as switching between each foot used to push off and generate momentum.

CIRCLE COUNTER-CLOCKWISE AND CLOCKWISE

Circling around the ring is one approach of retreating and creating space.

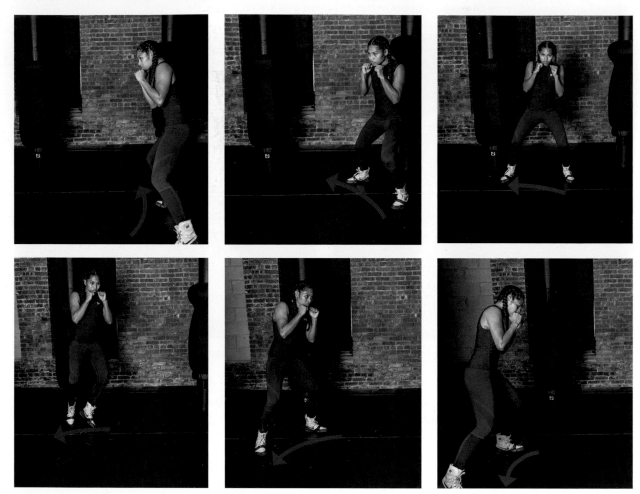

1. Push off one foot and keep your feet parallel to each other as you shuffle laterally in either a clockwise or counter-clockwise direction around the ring.

2. Practice moving and shifting in both directions, constantly changing the frequency and pace of each shift. Keep your hands in a neutral and ready position, ensuring your chin is protected as you move around.

CUTTING OFF THE RING

Understanding how to effectively control your target's movement around the ring gives you greater ability to control the pace of each exchange. Visualize the ring as being divided into four quadrants, with one corner in each quadrant. You will practice controlling the center of the ring. Your aim is to keep your target in one quadrant by cutting off their movement.

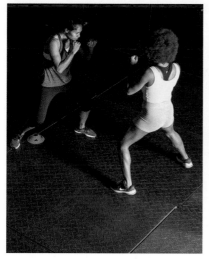 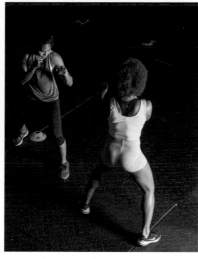 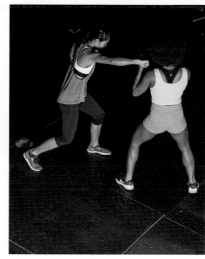

1. Begin in the center of the ring. Perceive your target stepping or moving to your right.

2. Take a step to the right with your right foot. Make sure that your step is wide enough so that your foot is on the outside of your perceived target's outermost foot. Adjust your left foot to bring yourself back into your neutral stance.

3. To add challenge to this exercise, throw a right hook as you step to the right to inhibit your perceived target from escaping.

4. Once your right foot steps to the outside of your perceived target's outermost foot, maintain control within the quadrant by pivoting on your rear foot to facilitate your lead foot lining up with your perceived target's center line. In other words, you want to make sure that your lead foot is splitting your perceived target into two equal halves.

5. Perceive your target stepping or moving to your left.

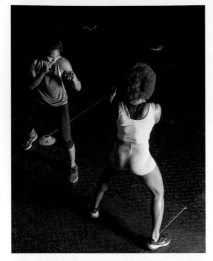 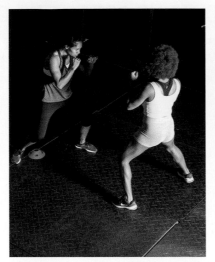 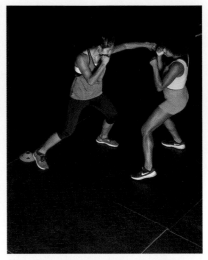

6. Take a step to the left with your left foot. Make sure that your step is wide enough so that your foot is on the outside of your perceived target's outermost foot. Adjust your right foot to bring yourself back into your neutral stance.

7. To add challenge to this exercise, throw a left hook as you step to the left to inhibit your perceived target from escaping.

8. Once your left foot steps to the outside of your perceived target's outermost foot, maintain control within the quadrant by pivoting on your rear foot to facilitate your lead foot lining up with your perceived target's center line. In other words, you want to make sure that your lead foot is splitting your perceived target into two equal halves.

9. Practice cutting off the ring by alternating steps to the right and left. After each step, try to pivot on your rear foot, making sure that your lead foot maintains a position that splits your perceived target into two equal halves.

DEFENSE

In the previous chapter, we examined the use of footwork to improve your connecting rate through specific movement and body mechanics. The proficient use of footwork is also conducive to building an effective defense. In this chapter, we will take a closer look at several defense methods used to minimize the impact of or avoid a punch altogether. The defensive techniques we will examine in this chapter include:

- Slipping punches
- Catch and throw
- Parrying
- Level changing

- Retreat and circling
- Retreat and counter
- Pivoting

SLIPPING PUNCHES

You can evade a barrage of punches with the effective use of slipping. There are several directions in which you can slip, and this often will depend on the angle from which a punch is thrown. For example, you might have a jab or cross thrown in a straight trajectory. To slip a straight punch you must take your head off the center line of attack by bending laterally around the waist. Typically, you would look to slip to the outside of a punch.

Let's use the example of two boxers with the same orthodox stance, i.e. the same left-foot lead. One boxer throws a jab while the other slips to the right (outside) of the punch. Because the boxer slips to the outside of the straight punch, he or she can counterpunch or escape without counterpunching.

In another possible scenario, the boxer slips to the left (inside) of the jab. In this scenario, the defensive boxer does not completely shift his or her head away from the line of attack, as the head is still within striking distance of a cross coming from the other boxer's rear hand. In this situation, the boxer has to follow up with an attack, typically a left hook to the body or head after slipping on the inside of the jab, in order to avoid a potential counterattack (cross) coming from the other boxer's rear hand.

These are a couple of tips to keep in mind when slipping:

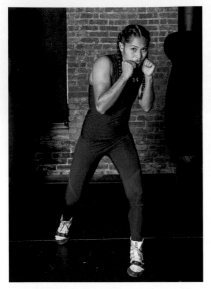
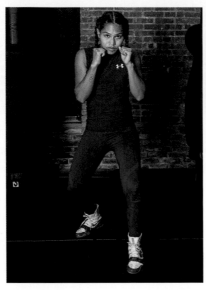
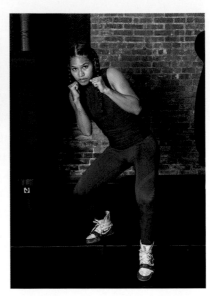

Take your hands with you: When you slip from one side to another, your hands should be level with and protecting your chin. Try not to drop your hands and expose your chin when you slip from side to side.

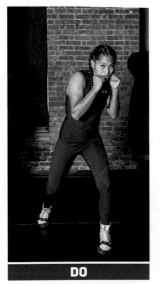
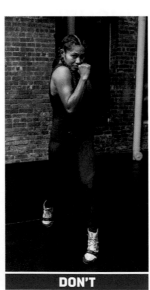
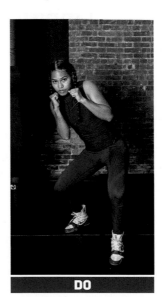
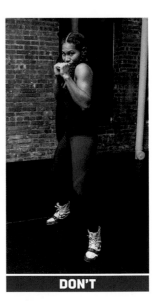

DO **DON'T** **DO** **DON'T**

Bend laterally around the waist as opposed to alternating and shifting your shoulders forward: Keep in mind that the objective of slipping is to take your head off the center line of attack. Alternating the shift of each shoulder forward and backward only slightly changes the distance between your head position and the center line of attack. Incorporating lateral bending around the waist helps create sufficient distance between your head position and the center line of attack.

We will cover more forms of slipping later in the chapter.

CATCH AND THROW

There are four ways to catch an incoming punch.

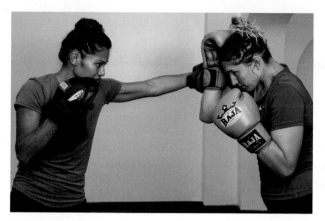
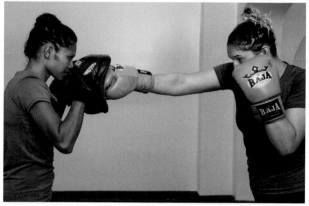

1. From your boxing stance, start by lifting your right shoulder to your ear, keeping your elbow tucked in. Make sure that your right hand stays pressed against the lateral aspect of your head. In this position, your arm serves as a protective shield and absorbs the impact of the punch. The same arm that catches the punch also throws the counterpunch; this could be a straight punch (jab or cross) or a right hook.

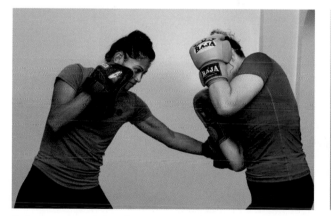
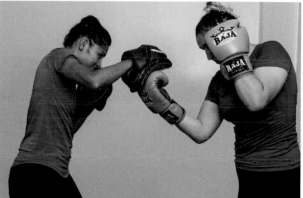

2. Lower your right elbow toward your hip to protect your body. Make sure that your right hand is tightly pressed against your chin. Again, the same arm that catches the punch throws the counterpunch; throw a right uppercut. You can also follow up with a left hook after throwing the counter right uppercut.

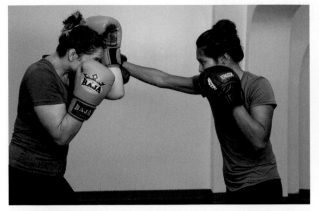 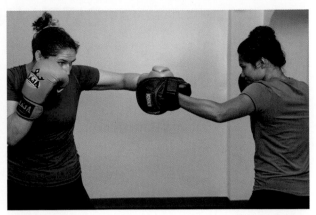

3. Lift your left shoulder to your ear, keeping your elbow tucked in. Make sure your left hand stays pressed against the lateral aspect of your head. Follow up with a counter left hook.

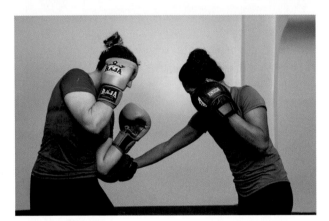 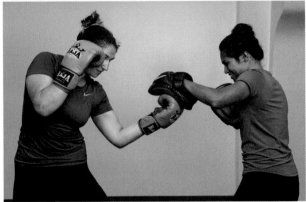

4. Lower your left elbow toward your hip to protect your body. Make sure that your left hand is tightly pressed against your chin. Follow up with a counter left uppercut and straight punch with your right hand.

Make sure there is minimal distance between your elbow, forearm, and lateral aspect of your waist when catching a punch. Do not reach away from your head or body to catch punches. This is counterproductive, as it would create distance between the elbow, forearm, and lateral aspect of your waist; if an incoming punch is powerful enough it could overpower your forearm, driving it backward and causing you to strike yourself.

PARRYING

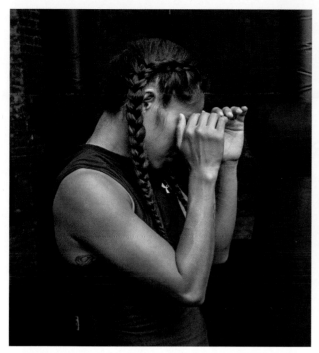 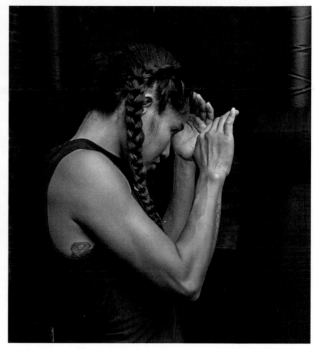

When you parry a punch, you deflect the incoming force of a punch away from you. Without reaching toward the punch, you want to create just enough tension in your arm to prevent the impact of the punch from changing the inner angle of your elbow. Additionally, rotate your wrist so that the palm of your hand parries the punch downward and away from your face. You can make this more challenging by adding steps, pivoting, circling, and counterpunches to your parries. Practice the parries below:

- Parry with the rear hand and counter with a jab
- Parry with the lead hand and counter with a cross
- Parry with the lead hand and pivot to the left
- Parry with the right hand pivoting to the right

LEVEL CHANGING

Think about how difficult it is to hit a moving target. Boxing utilizes movement as a method to help maneuver a moving target to a desired position for an offensive attack and to create an elusive form of defense.

Level changing is movement that occurs when you adjust your height by changing the inner angle of your knee joint. This ascending and descending movement inhibits attacks because it is quite challenging to connect punches to a target in perpetual motion.

RETREAT

Retreat and Circling: To retreat, push off your lead foot to step backward and away from an incoming punch. When you have successfully cleared the punch using the initial retreat step, make sure that your feet are parallel to each other, which will allow you to shuffle your feet as you continue to circle around the ring or space in either a clockwise or a counterclockwise direction. (See page 32 for circling.) Develop good defense habits by keeping your chin protected as you move around.

Retreat and Counter: When you retreat (step back), you must push off your lead foot and step backward to avoid an incoming punch. You are now in a safer position to throw a counterpunch. Practice some counterpunching combinations:

- Retreat and counter with a cross

- Retreat and counter with a cross/lead hook

- Retreat and counter with a jab/cross

- Retreat and counter with a jab/cross/lead hook

- Retreat and counter with a rear uppercut

- Retreat and counter with a rear uppercut/lead hook

PIVOTING

You can avoid a flurry or barrage of punches by moving away from the line of attack. Pivoting is one method of moving away from the line of attack. (See page 31 for tips on pivoting.) Practice pivoting with a counter.

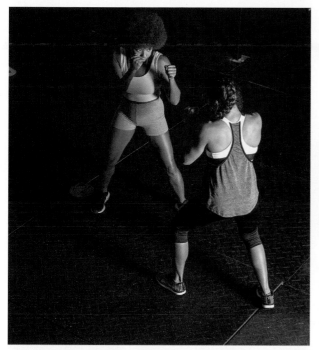 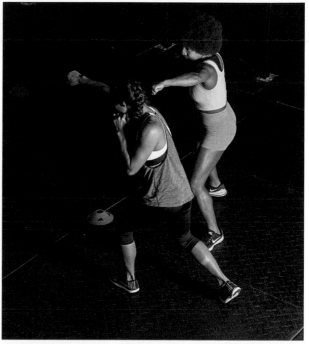

1. Starting in your neutral stance, step with your lead foot and then rotate on the ball of your lead foot as you simultaneously throw a hook with your lead hand. This technique is called a "check hook."

2. You can double up on the check hook as you pivot by throwing one hook to the lateral side of the target's head and then following up with a second hook to the lateral side of the target's body.

DEFENSIVE EXERCISES

The following exercises will help you apply the defensive techniques covered in this chapter. Practice a defense drill by combining the following techniques: Slip Side to Side, Dip, Pull Back, Pivot 180 Degrees, and Weave Side to Side.

SLIP SIDE TO SIDE

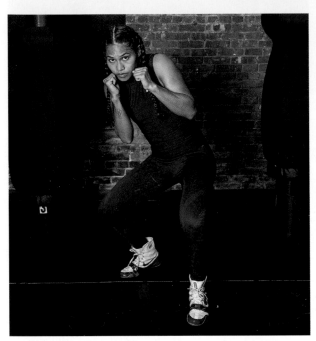 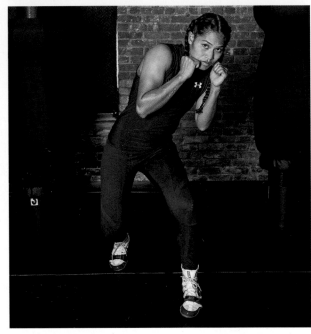

1. Slip to the side adjacent to your rear foot by bending laterally around the waist to shift your head position away from the center line of attack.

2. Point your rear knee away from the lead foot as you lower your level. Make sure that you take your hands with you throughout this movement; your hands should constantly protect your chin.

3. Slip in the opposite direction. Slightly pivot on the ball of your rear foot as you lower your level and bend laterally around the waist to shift your head position away from the center line of attack. Your hips should be square in front of the target with both knees pointing forward. Make sure that your hands protect your chin throughout the entire motion. This action helps protect against any straight punches, such as the jab and cross.

DIP

You are level changing in this exercise.

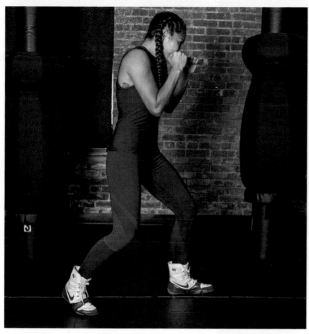 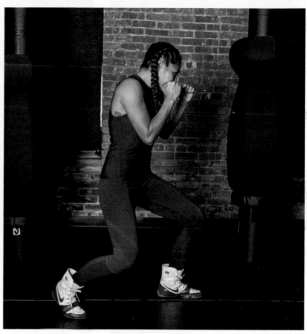

1. Keep your hands by your chin as you quickly lower your level by bending your knees. Keep the inner angle of the knee greater than or equal to 90 degrees.

2. Extend your knees to return to the initial position.

PULL BACK

1. Keeping your lead foot in place, take a step back on the rear foot.

2. Lean your weight backward to avoid incoming punches.

3. Once punches are cleared, step the rear foot back into your starting position.

PIVOT 180 DEGREES

Push off your rear foot to generate forward momentum, which you will redirect as you pivot on the ball of your lead foot to change the direction you are facing by 180 degrees.

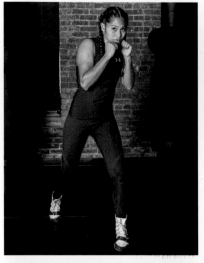 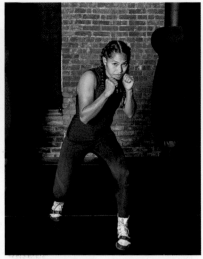 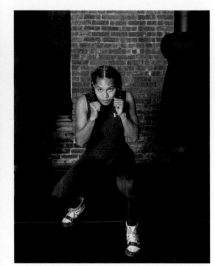

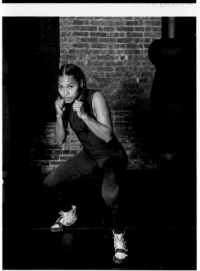 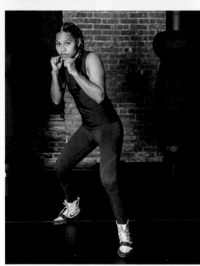

1. Keeping your hands by your chin for protection, lower your level as you rotate around the waist to the side adjacent to your rear foot.

2. Your head position should be away from the center line as you return to normal level.

3. Weave to the other side by lowering your level and rotating at the waist to the side adjacent to your lead foot.

4. Again, your head position should be away from the center line as you return to normal level. From start to finish, you are making the shape of a "U" with this movement.

Note: Make sure that you are bouncing as you transition between these defensive techniques to practice coordination and rhythm. If you have a rope available, you can set it up to run from one end of the room to the other. Start in your boxing stance and practice weaving back and forth from one end of the rope to the other.

BOXING MECHANICS

Understanding muscle recruitment and body mechanics plays an essential role in building your level of proficiency in boxing for fitness. This section examines several important concepts, including:

1. Effective punching technique

2. Generating power through speed

3. Muscular endurance

4. Balance and stability

5. Self-correcting adjustments

6. Shadowboxing exercises

EFFECTIVE PUNCHING TECHNIQUE

A punch aims to deliver force to a specific location on a desired target, which requires energy and effort. The effectiveness of that punch is measured by how much of the generated force, ideally the maximum impact, is absorbed by the target. When the arm extends to connect a closed and turned fist to a target, the effectiveness of that punch is contingent upon whether any amount of the generated force is dispersed around the target. In other words, a punch becomes less effective if only a fraction of the maximum impact is absorbed by the target. This could be caused by several impeding factors. One obvious factor is that your target effectively blocks the punch. Another factor, and the primary focus of this section, is on how you deliver the punch using proper mechanics to develop a higher level of accuracy.

To better understand, let's start with a simple exercise as a basis of reference. Get into your boxing stance so that your dominant hand throws a cross. When ready, throw a cross and keep your arm extended. Take note of your position here.

At the end of this punch, you might notice one of three things:

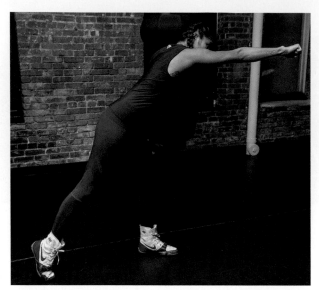

You are leaning too far over your lead foot: This is also known as overextending and "falling forward" in the direction of your target. This also causes being off balance. While some of the force is absorbed by the target upon connecting, the impact and power of the punch is reduced. This is because active tension in your forward-leaning body causes you to reach the target more slowly; it is an inefficient use of energy and effort.

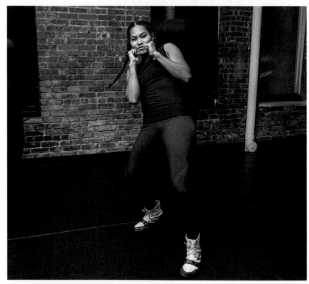

You are leaning too far back on your rear foot, or simply, "leaning back": This form of being off-balance occurs when you lean your weight backward over the rear foot, away from the direction of your target. While some of the force is absorbed by the target upon connecting, the impact and power of the punch is reduced. This is because the active tension in your backward-leaning body pulls some of the power away from the target, also causing you to reach the target more slowly.

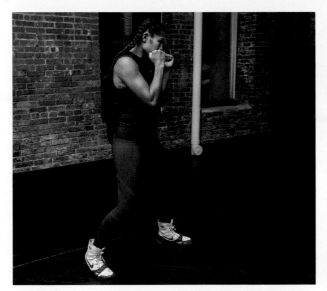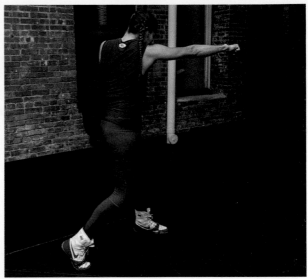

Your weight is equally centered over both feet: In this instance, you are in a balanced and ideal position to deliver the full power of your punch to the desired target. Transferring the generated force of your punch so that the target absorbs the maximum impact is achieved through extension of the elbow, rotation around the wrist and waist, and pivoting of the rear foot. No energy is wasted in this scenario, as every movement has a direct purpose relevant to delivering an effective punch. No incremental work must be done to regain balance and stabilize the body; therefore, every movement is precisely calculated to achieve the highest level of efficiency when throwing the punch.

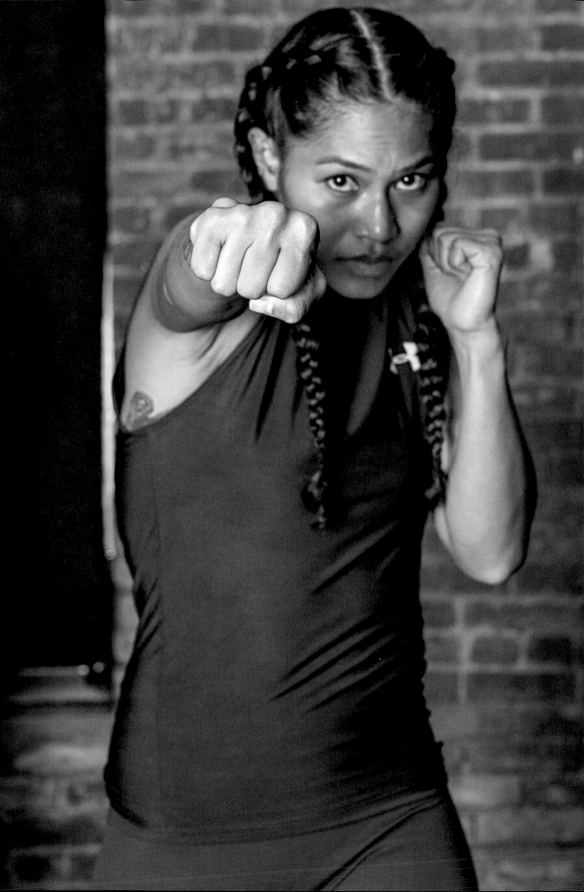

Let's do a similar exercise using a different punch. Get into your boxing stance. When ready, throw a lead hook and hold your position.

At the end of this punch, you might notice any of the following:

- The end of your closed fist is past the center line of your chin

- You are over-rotating and moving past your target

- You are leaning too far over your lead foot

- You are pulling and leaning backward on your rear foot

When any of the above occur, the impact of the placement of your punch on a physical or perceived stationary target mirroring your position decreases, as some of the generated force is dispersed around your desired target. Ideally, when punching, the effort in muscle recruitment stops upon immediate connection to your physical or perceived target. Following the connection of your punch is the effort in retraction. Any additional effort exerted to further extend your punch after you make a connection results in the inefficient use of energy, which transfers force of impact around, instead of directly and solely on, a target.

GENERATING POWER THROUGH SPEED

According to the third edition of the *NASM Essentials of Personal Fitness Training*, power is defined as the ability of the neuromuscular system to produce the greatest force in the shortest time. To illustrate this concept, let's use the example of a tire flip exercise. As you begin to lift the tire, you must exert enough energy to move the object. The use of strength, which the same book defines as the ability of the neuromuscular system to provide internal tension and exert force against an external resistance, acts as the resisting force against the weight of the tire. As the tire drops in the latter portion of the exercise there is no external resistance against its falling weight until it hits the floor.

Despite the equal distance between the highest possible vertical point of the tire and the floor, there is a clear distinction in the resulting impact on the tire. In the upward trajectory, the unequal and opposite tension between the weight of the tire and the resisting force (strength) causes the object to move in the direction it is being pushed. The impact in this scenario is low, as the force against the tire pushes the object at a much slower speed despite the strength generated to influence this effect. In the downward trajectory, the absence of a resisting force (strength) against the weight of the tire causes the object to accelerate. As the tire hits the floor (the resisting force), the force of the impact is high because the tire collides against the floor with an accelerated speed that ends abruptly.

In boxing, you can generate power through speed. A fist weighs far less than the rest of your body and therefore can reach the target much quicker if supported by the proper body mechanics. Your hips generate a great amount of power as proximal and larger muscles in your legs and buttocks produce strength. Through rotation of the hip and extension of the arm, speed is produced and your punch travels at a high velocity until it connects with the desired target. Upon connecting with the target, the acceleration of your punch stops abruptly due to the sudden presence of a resisting force, i.e. your target, and in this exact moment, the force of the impact is high.

You must retract your arm after your target absorbs the maximum impact of your punch. Doing so not only ensures you keep a strong defense to protect yourself, which is a good habit to develop, but also effectively resets you back into a balanced and neutral stance to execute additional punches.

MUSCULAR ENDURANCE

Developing muscular endurance through repetitive motion against a resisting force helps improve defensive and offensive efficiency. Boxing requires periodic use of muscle relaxation to create efficient movement as well as tension to inhibit opposing force. Managing the application of both relaxation and tension allows the body to develop a level of muscular endurance needed to maintain balance, increase output, and maintain an effective guard through retraction. Balance, output, and retraction efficiency all serve as visual measurements of one's overall endurance level.

During periods of relaxation, the body can utilize speed and range of motion to create efficient movement. This is particularly useful when throwing punches. Tension must be applied upon impact to transfer the generated force and prevent overextension.

There are many endurance exercises that simulate the pace and intensity found in boxing. Endurance exercises on the following pages can be incorporated into your training regimen.

SHADOWBOXING WITH WEIGHTS

1. Begin shadowboxing holding a pair of 2-pound or 5-pound weights. Focus on maintaining proper form and keeping the trajectory of the punches as you would without the added weight. Shadowbox for 3 minutes per round for 3 rounds.

2. Put the weights down and continue to shadowbox, focusing on speed for the last 30 seconds of each round. Your primary focus here is to maintain your balance, composure, and technique by slowing the punches down when fatigue starts to set in.

ROTATIONAL SINGLE-ARM PRESS WITH LANDMINE

If your gym does not have a landmine, you can improvise by placing one end of a barbell in the corner of the wall.

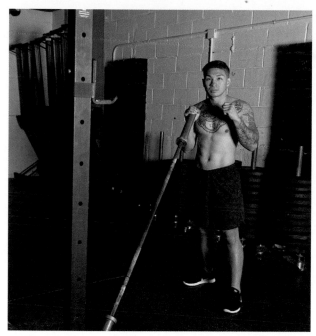 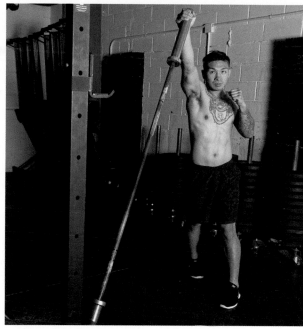

1. Start in a neutral stance, holding one end of the barbell with a relaxed grip and resting your other hand at your shoulder.

2. Extend your arm, keeping your back straight, and pivot your rear foot so that your toes are facing forward. Make sure that your extended arm, back, and rear leg are all aligned.

3. Lower the barbell, moving into a staggered squat, with feet shoulder-width apart and your rear foot about a foot behind the lead foot.

Repeat the exercise 8 to 10 times, alternating each arm for 3 sets.

SQUAT WITH LANDMINE

If your gym does not have a landmine, you can improvise by placing one end of a barbell in the corner of the wall.

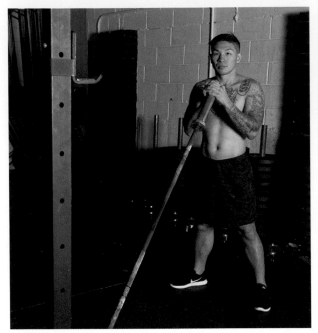 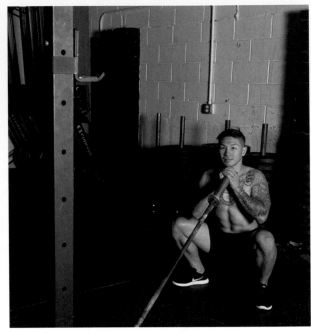

1. Start with your feet shoulder-width apart, holding the barbell by your chest with both hands.

2. Lower your body into a deep squat with your knees pointed outward as you descend until you have about a 90-degree angle in both knees. Keep your head up, back angled slightly forward but straight, elbows tucked, chest out, and hips square.

3. Extend both legs to bring yourself back to starting position.

Repeat the exercise 8 to 10 times for 3 sets.

THRUSTER WITH LANDMINE

If your gym does not have a landmine, you can improvise by placing one end of a barbell in the corner of the wall.

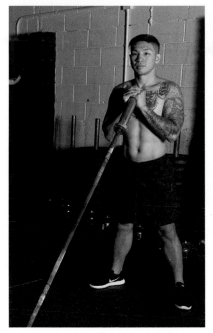 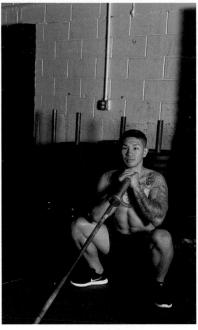 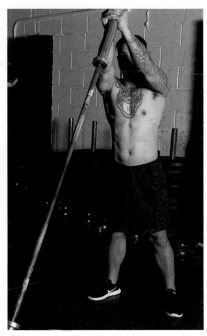

1. Start with your feet parallel and shoulder-width apart, holding the barbell by your chest with both hands.

2. Lower your body into a deep squat, pointing your knees outward as you descend, until you have about a 90-degree angle in both knees. You may descend into a deeper squat if you have that range of motion. Keep your head up and back angled slightly forward but straight, with your elbows tucked, chest out, and hips square.

3. Extend both legs as well as arms as you ascend. Both arms should be extended above your head.

Repeat the exercise 8 to 10 times for 3 sets.

ANTI-ROTATION WITH LANDMINE

If your gym does not have a landmine, you can improvise by placing one end of a barbell in the corner of the wall.

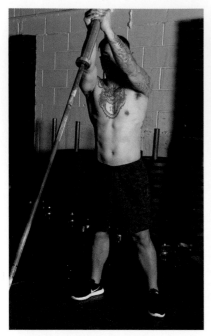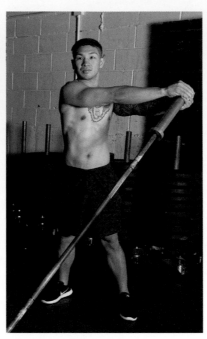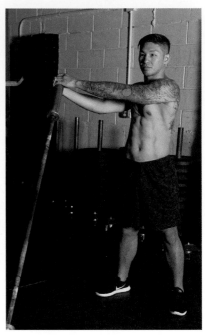

1. Start with your feet shoulder-width apart. Hold the end of the barbell with both hands. Keep your arms straight without rotating your hips or shoulders.

2. Move the bar in a semi-spherical motion from one side to the other, keeping your arms straight throughout the entire motion.

Repeat the exercise 8 to 10 times for 3 sets.

MEADOW'S ROW WITH LANDMINE

If your gym does not have a landmine, you can improvise by placing one end of a barbell in the corner of the wall.

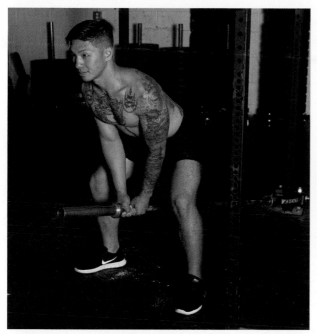 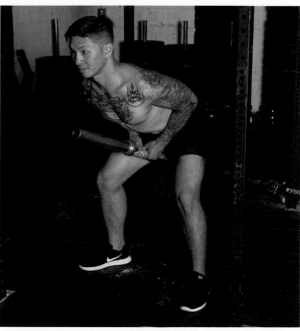

1. Stand over the barbell holding one end of it with both hands. Keep your feet shoulder-width apart with the end of the barbell resting at your center line.

2. Keeping your back straight, bend forward around the waist to sit in a high squat, to hold the end of the barbell with the nearest arm.

3. Pull the barbell into your chest area and control the weight of the barbell as you extend your arm out.

Repeat the exercise 8 to 10 times, alternating each arm for 3 sets.

SINGLE-ARM PUSH PRESS WITH LANDMINE

If your gym does not have a landmine, you can improvise by placing one end of a barbell in the corner of the wall.

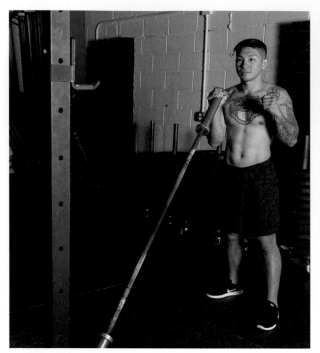 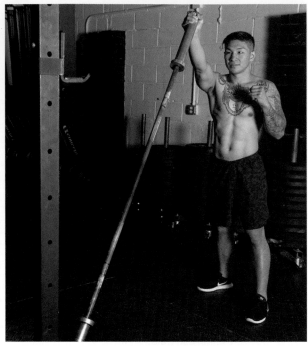

1. Stand with your feet shoulder-width apart, holding one end of the barbell with a relaxed grip and resting your other hand at your shoulder.

2. Press the barbell upward, extending your arm.

3. Return to starting position.

Repeat the exercise 8 to 10 times, alternating each arm for 3 sets.

SINGLE-ARM PUSH PRESS SWITCHES WITH LANDMINE

If your gym does not have a landmine, you can improvise by placing one end of a barbell in the corner of the wall.

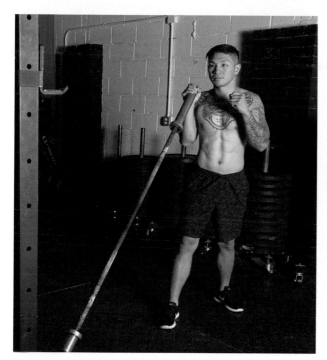 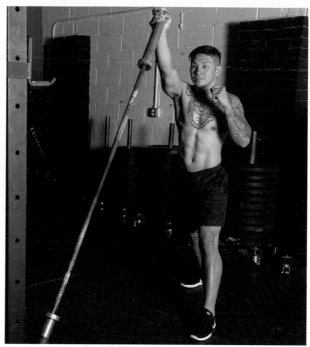

1. Start in a neutral stance, holding one end of the barbell with a relaxed grip and resting your other hand at your shoulder.

2. Shuffle your feet to switch your stance as you extend your arm to press the barbell upward.

3. Shuffle your feet to switch back to your starting stance as you lower the barbell back to resting position by your shoulder.

Repeat the exercise 8 to 10 times, alternating each arm for 3 sets.

PUSH-UP

You can incorporate Pull-Ups (page 59) and Dips (page 60) in between sets to complement this exercise and add variety and challenge to your regimen.

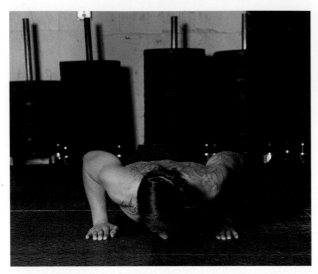 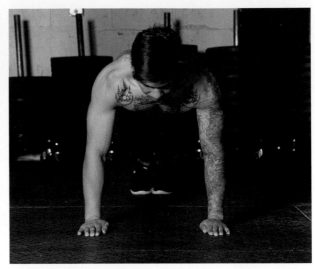

1. Keep your hands shoulder-width apart, your back straight, head aligned with your body, and core engaged. Lower your chest toward the floor.

2. As you push-up, make sure that you keep your core engaged and your back straight. As you extend your arms to complete the push-up, avoid arching your lower back by dropping or leaving your hips low to the floor.

Repeat the exercise 10 times for 3 sets.

PULL-UP

You can add Push-Ups (page 58) and Dips (page 60) in between sets to complement this exercise and add variety and challenge to your regimen.

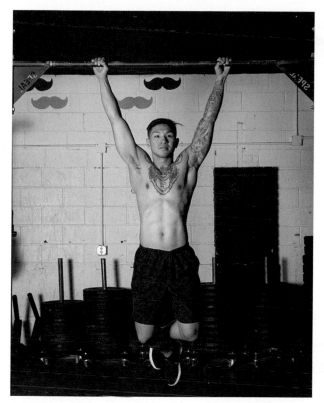 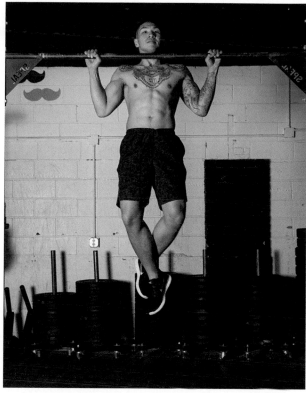

1. Grip the pull-up bar so that your palms are facing outward and away from you.

2. Engage your core and latissimus dorsi muscles as you pull yourself up toward the bar. Make sure that your chin clears the bar before extending your arms and lowering yourself back to your starting position.

Repeat the exercise 10 times for 3 sets.

DIP

If you do not have access to a dip machine, you can improvise and use a chair or bench as an alternative. You can add Push-Ups (page 58) and Pull-Ups (page 59) in between sets to complement this exercise and add variety and challenge to your regimen.

If using a dip machine:

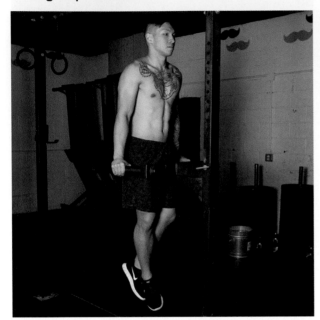 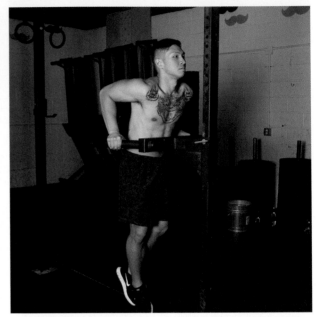

1. Start with arms extended and both hands gripping each of the dip bars.

2. Keep your knees bent and your shoulders and core engaged as you descend, stopping when you've reached a 90-degree angle in your elbows.

3. Extend your arms to push and bring yourself back to your starting position.

Repeat this exercise 10 times for 3 sets.

If using a chair or bench:

1. Start with arms extended and both hands about shoulder-width apart, placed palm-down on the bench. Make sure that your buttocks are off the bench.

2. Keep your legs relaxed with a slight bend in your knees (alternatively you can keep your legs relaxed and extended).

3. Engage your shoulders and core as you descend your body, stopping when you've reached a 90-degree angle in your elbows.

4. Extend your arms to push and bring yourself back to your starting position.

Repeat this exercise 10 times for 3 sets.

CHIN-UP TO PULL-UP

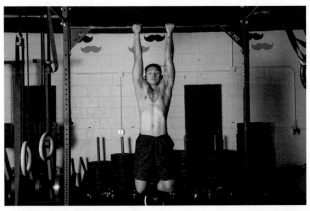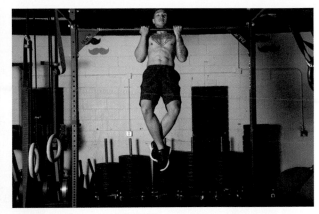

1. Begin with both hands gripping the bar with palms facing inward toward you. Engage your core and biceps to pull your chin up to the bar. Your chin should clear the bar.

2. Extend your arms and lower yourself back to your starting position.

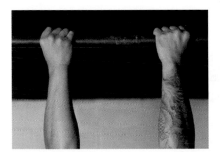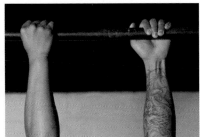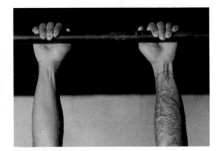

3. Switch your grip, one hand at a time, so that your palms face outward and away from you.

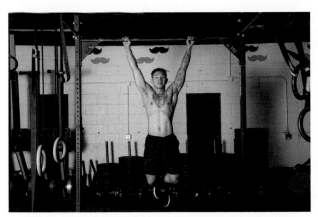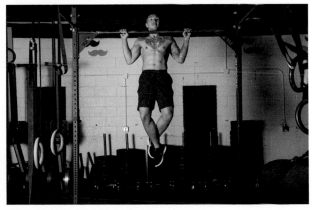

4. Engage your core and latissimus dorsi muscles as you pull yourself up toward the bar. Make sure that your chin clears the bar before extending your arms and lowering yourself back to your starting position.

Switch between chin-ups and pull-ups 8 to 10 times for 3 sets.

JUMP SQUAT

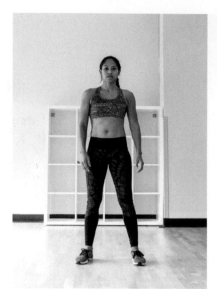 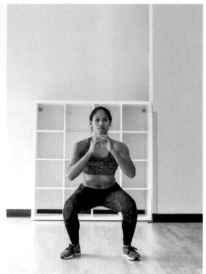 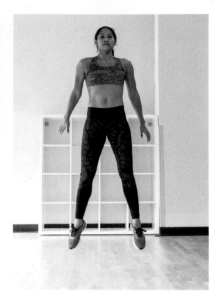

1. Stand upright, with your feet slightly wider than shoulder width. Keep your arms relaxed and extended down the length of your body.

2. Lower yourself into a deep squat, with knees bent at about a 90-degree angle and pointed outward. Keep your head up, your chest out, and your hips square. Curl your arms in toward your body as you lower into the squat. Push off your feet in an explosive vertical jump, extending your arms down the length of your body.

3. Upon landing, lower into a deep squat to repeat previous motion.

Repeat the full cycle of this exercise from starting position 8 to 10 times for 3 sets.

BOSU BALL JUMP SQUAT

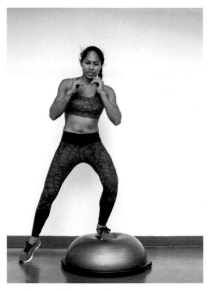 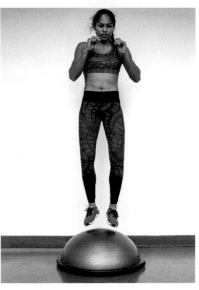 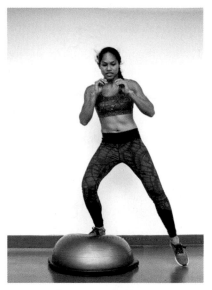

1. Start with one foot on the center of the BOSU ball, keeping your spine in alignment and arms curled in to your body. Your other foot is placed on the floor. Keep your feet parallel.

2. Keep your head up, your back angled slightly forward but straight, elbows tucked, chest out, and hips square as you lower yourself into a squat.

3. Explode into a vertical jump over the BOSU ball as you switch out the foot on the center of the ball and lower yourself back into a squat position.

Repeat, alternating sides 20 times per foot for 4 sets.

TREADMILL SPRINTS

1. Warm up at a moderate speed for 1 to 1¹/₂ miles. Then, adjust to highest incline.

2. Sprint uphill on highest incline for 30 seconds. Rest for 30 seconds.

Repeat the last step for 10 sprints (10 minutes). Adjust the sprints according to your level of fitness:

- Beginner: sprint 10 seconds; rest 20 seconds. 10 total sprints (5 minutes)

- Intermediate: sprint 20 seconds; rest 10 seconds. 10 total sprints (5 minutes)

- Experienced: sprint 30 seconds; rest 30 seconds. 10 total sprints (10 minutes)

HEAVY BAG DRILL

You will need an interval timer for this drill. Set the timer for a 1-minute work round with a 10-second rest period in between rounds. You will drill for 10 rounds total.

1. When the timer sounds for the first minute, throw power shot hooks (heavy punches with maximum force) to the body of the heavy bag.

2. When the timer sounds for the second minute, switch to nonstop straight punches (jab and cross).

Straight punches are meant to focus on quickness and speed, so do not load up on power when throwing these punches.

Alternate between power shots and nonstop straight punches every round.

JUMP ROPE AND DOUBLE-UNDER JUMPS

You will need a boxing bell timer for this exercise. Set the timer for a 3-minute round with a 1-minute rest period in between rounds. You will complete 3 rounds.

1. Start jumping when the bell sounds.

2. Switch to double-under jumps when the rest bell sounds. Double-under jumps require more air time, as the rope travels under your feet twice in one repetition. Make sure that you keep your legs fully extended, and slightly kick both feet in front of you by bending at the waist when you jump.

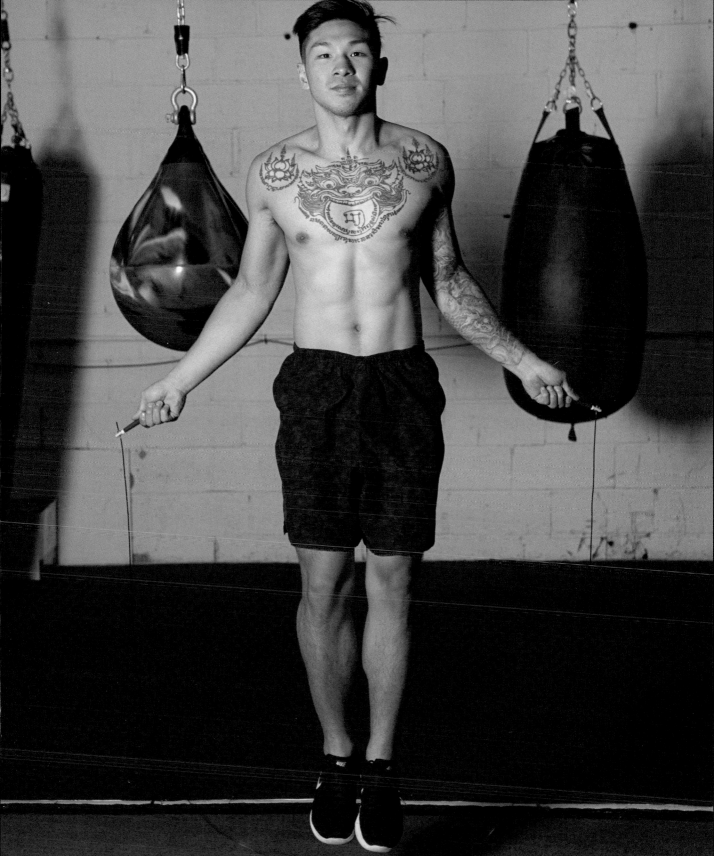

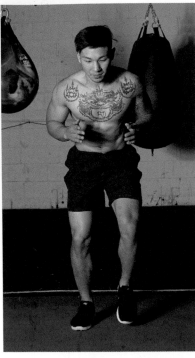 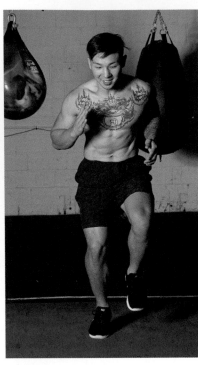 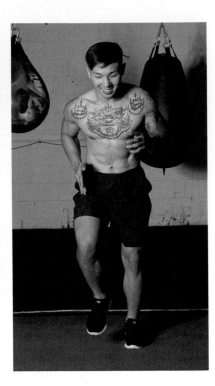

1. Stand with your feet parallel and shoulder-width apart.

2. Keep your weight on the balls of your feet as you run in place.

3. Alternate lifting each foot off the floor as quickly as you can. Your objective is to minimize the amount of time in between lifting and returning (maximizing the number of repetitions of) each foot to the floor.

Tip: Maintain a position with a slight bend in your knees and chest leaning forward so that your shoulders are directly over your knees. This position helps improve your speed as it requires only a partial degree of change in the angle of your knee that you need in order to lift your foot off the floor. A more upright position with no bend in the knees would require a greater degree of change in the angle of the knee, which adds more time to your overall performance.

QUICK FEET TO SPRAWL

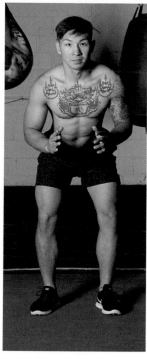 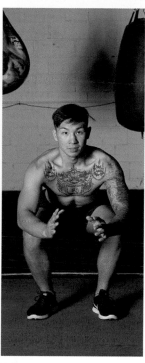 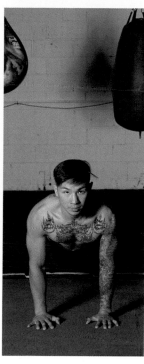 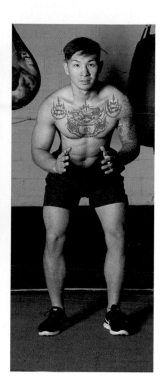

1. Perform Quick Feet (page 66) for 5 to 10 seconds, then sprawl.

2. To sprawl, bend at the waist as you extend your arms downward, placing both hands on the floor.

3. Kick your feet backward so that you end up in push-up position. (It is acceptable to allow your hips to sink close to the floor during a sprawl.)

4. Immediately push off your feet to bring your knees up toward your chest and to return your feet under your hips. Quickly return to your standing position.

JUMPING LUNGE

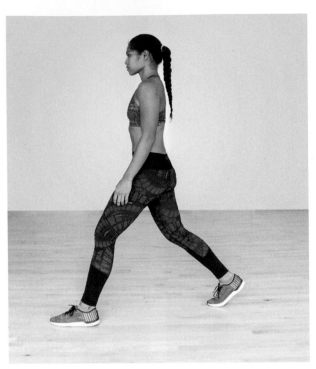 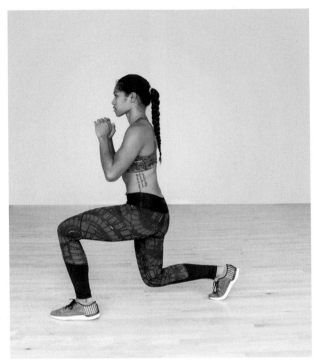

1. Stand with feet shoulder-width apart.

2. Step one foot forward and lower yourself into a deep lunge. Make sure you have about a 90-degree angle in your knees and your rear knee is just off the floor.

3. Keep your hands rested on your hips as you explode into a vertical jump and land back into lunge position.

Do 20 jumping lunges per side for a total of 40 jumping lunges for 3 sets.

KICK-BACK BURPEE TO PLANK PUSH-UP

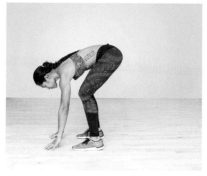
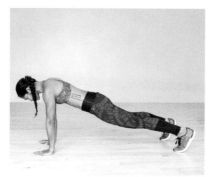
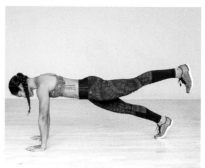
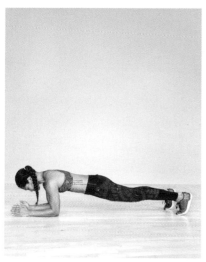
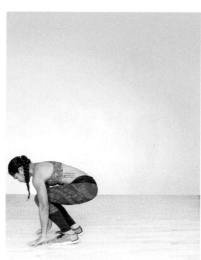
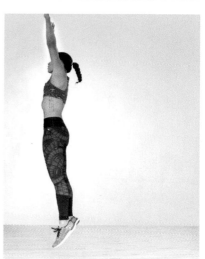

1. Stand upright and bend at the waist to bring your hands to the floor. Once your hands are on the floor and stable, kick your feet back so that you end up in push-up position.

2. Keeping your legs extended, lift your left leg as far up as your range of motion will allow. Repeat this motion with the right leg. Return to push-up position.

3. From push-up position, lower one elbow to the floor, then the other. Keeping your core engaged, place one hand on the floor, then the other, and extend your arm to push your body up.

4. Quickly bring your feet under your hips and jump up with explosive power as you extend your arms upward, as if to reach for the ceiling. End in a standing position.

Repeat the full cycle of this exercise from starting position for 1 minute.

MOUNTAIN CLIMBER BURPEE

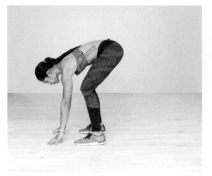
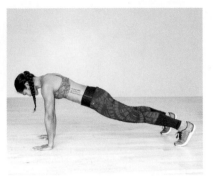
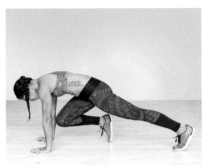

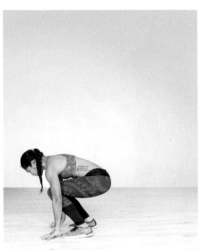
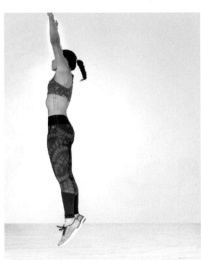

1. Stand upright and bend at the waist to bring your hands to the floor. Once your hands are on the floor and stable, kick your feet back so that you end up in push-up position.

2. Do two mountain climbers. To perform one repetition, quickly and smoothly bring one knee upward toward the chest, return the leg to the ground, then repeat with your other knee.

3. Now immediately bring your feet under your hips and jump up with explosive power as you extend your arms upward, as if to reach for the ceiling. End in a standing position.

Repeat the full cycle of this exercise from starting position for 1 minute.

BALANCE AND STABILITY

As you train and execute various techniques, maintaining balance not only indicates an increased level of endurance but also yields a higher rate of efficiency. When balanced, your body consistently resets to its neutral stance, and any unnecessary motion is eliminated. Unnecessary motion negatively affects the timing, impact, and effectiveness of a technique.

To illustrate an example of unnecessary motion, we will use a simple combination of the jab and cross. Standing in neutral stance, you throw the jab and cross twice for a total of four punches. Before the initial punch is thrown, you are standing in neutral stance with hands protecting the chin and elbows protecting your body. You then extend the first punch, a jab, followed by the second punch, a cross. Now, in the return of each punch you retract your hands around the chest area, rather than to the chin. The second time the jab and cross are thrown, you must make certain adjustments before extending the set of punches, as resetting to a non-neutral stance changes the trajectory of the punches, effectively reducing the overall impact of the punches. First, your defense is compromised because your hands are resting by your chest, leaving your chin exposed. Second, adjusting to bring your hands up to chin level adds to the amount of time it will take for your punch to reach your intended target.

As a rule of thumb, you want to return to neutral stance after each attack to maintain a strong defense and efficient offensive output. Returning to your neutral stance after an attack, whether you are the one countering an attack or initiating to advance an attack, keeps the level of stability required to maintain balance and a strong defense.

One of the best ways to ensure that you maintain balance and stability is to be aware of your center of gravity. Be mindful of where your hips are in relation to your feet. Standing in neutral stance, notice that your hips should be between both feet. Self-check to make sure that you are not leaning too far forward or too far backward. A clear indicator that you are leaning too far forward is when you can lift your rear foot off the floor while standing in neutral stance. That indicates that all your weight is shifted over the lead foot. Conversely, leaning too far backward occurs when you can lift your lead foot off the floor while standing in neutral stance. This indicates that all your weight is shifted over the rear foot. Leaning too far forward or backward makes you susceptible to getting pushed over by a target whose center of gravity is kept in control. If you lean too far forward, you also face a higher chance of getting counterpunched, and if you lean too far backward, you may find it difficult to counter, as you may not be within punching range.

You can practice the following drills with a partner to develop balance and stability, which is especially difficult to maintain when moving around.

ANGLE OFF USING SIDE STEP AND PIVOT

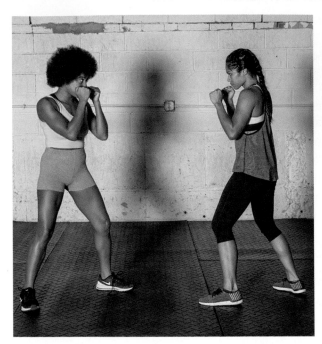 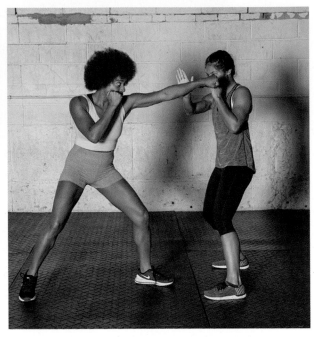

1. Standing in neutral stance with your partner facing you, advance and slowly extend a jab and cross. Your partner will step in the direction adjacent to his or her lead foot and pivot 90 degrees to avoid getting hit.

2. Switch roles so that it is now your partner's turn to advance, and slowly extend the jab and cross. As your partner advances, take a step in the direction adjacent to your lead foot and pivot 90 degrees to avoid getting run into.

Practice this drill while being mindful of keeping your center of gravity in control and maintaining your balance. Aim to return to neutral stance as you move around.

SHOULDER TAP

This is an effective drill that helps you learn to gauge, measure, and adjust how big or small of a step you need to take to be out of range as attacks are initiated, but to quickly step within range to deliver your own counterpunches. This is especially challenging because you must be moving on your feet while maintaining your balance and stability such that your center of gravity is controlled as you do so.

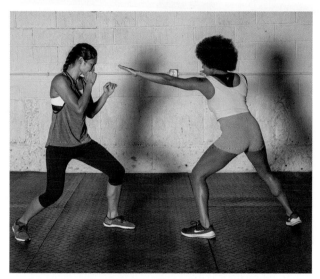 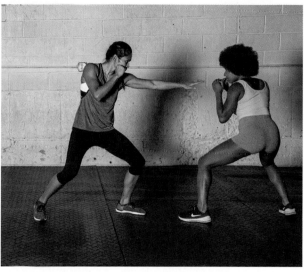

1. Standing in neutral stance with your partner facing you, take two steps forward, extending your jab to quickly and lightly tap your partner's lead shoulder. As you step forward, your partner retreats to avoid contact.

2. Your partner will then counter by taking two steps forward, extending his or her jab to quickly and lightly tap your lead shoulder. As your partner advances, you should be retreating to avoid contact.

Practice this drill back and forth with your partner for 3 minutes per round for 3 rounds.

HAND-TO-TOE CRUNCH

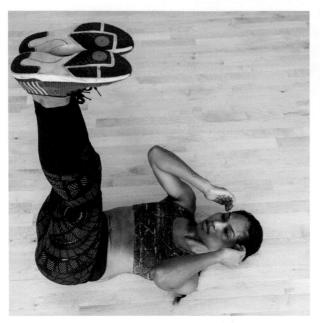 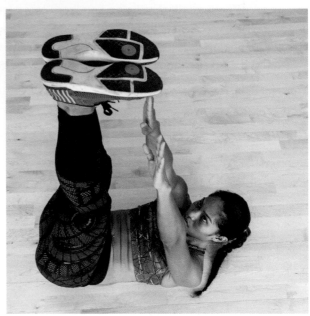

1. Lay on your back with your legs extended vertically.

2. Keep your legs extended as you engage your core and reach to touch your toes.

3. Bring your hands toward your face as you relax your core, keeping both legs extended.

Do 50 total repetitions.

ELBOW-TO-KNEE CRUNCH

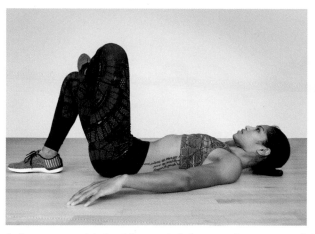 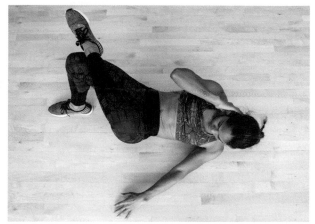

1. Lay on your back with your left foot resting on your right knee. Bend your right arm with your fingers placed by your right ear.

2. Engage your core and bring your right elbow toward your left knee. Relax your core as you bring your right elbow back to the starting position. Repeat this motion 25 times.

Switch sides and repeat another 25 times.

PULSE CRUNCH

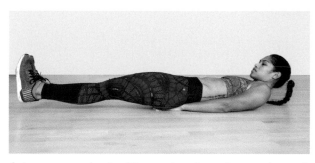 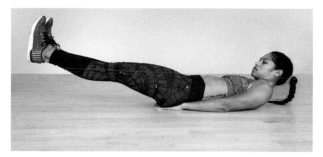

1. Lay on your back with your hands under your buttocks. Lift your head slightly off the floor and look toward your feet. Keep your feet off the floor.

2. Engage your core and lift your feet 6 to 8 inches off the floor. Lower your feet without touching the floor.

Do 50 total repetitions.

360-DEGREE ABS

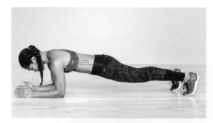 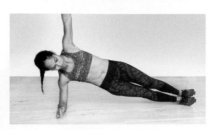 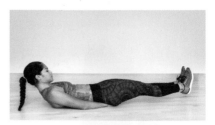

1. Start in a raised push-up position, with your arms extended, and lower into a plank position, with your elbows and forearms on the floor. Hold this position for 30 seconds.

2. Without lowering your hip to the floor, rotate into side plank while maintaining balance on your elbow and on the sides of your feet. Keep your spine aligned and core engaged. Hold this position for 30 seconds.

3. Rotate to lie with your back on the floor. Place your hands under your buttocks and lift your feet just off the floor. Engage your core and lift your head, keeping your chin tucked in to maintain a visual of your feet. Hold this position for 30 seconds.

4. Rotate into side plank on the other side. Maintain your balance on your elbow and on the sides of your feet. Keep your spine aligned and core engaged. Hold this position for 30 seconds.

5. Rotate into plank position. Keep your spine aligned and look forward. Without sinking your hips, keep your core engaged and hold this position for 30 seconds.

Do 3 complete 360-degree rotations.

SELF-CORRECTING ADJUSTMENTS

Knowing when and what to self-correct is beneficial to improving your overall offensive and defensive skill. Learn to identify factors that could potentially become problematic. Some of the more common beginner mistakes are listed on the following pages. Bear in mind that this list certainly does not cover all possible mistakes.

Over-rotating: Excessive rotation of the waist results in an off-balance stance, an inefficient use of energy to push a resisting force, and a compromised defense. A prime example of over-rotating occurs commonly when throwing hooks. As a rule of thumb, use your chin as the end point of a hook. In other words, the punch stops at your chin; your knuckles should be in line with your chin. Once your knuckles move past the line of your chin, you are over-rotating around the waist.

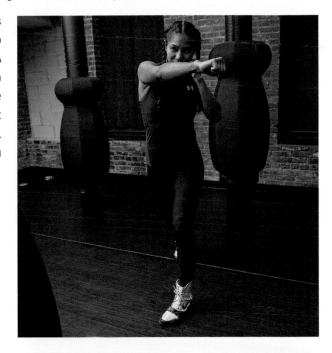

Overextending: Excessive extension of the arm results in an off-balance stance and may also cause overreaching. When you overreach, you essentially lean your body too far forward over your feet, which compromises your defense and leaves you susceptible to easily being counterpunched.

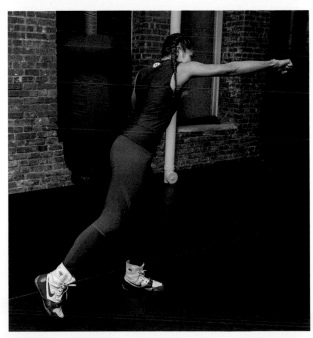

Telegraphing punches: In boxing, telegraphing means allowing your opponent to easily anticipate your next move through certain pre-adjustments made to your neutral stance prior to execution. Telegraphing, or winding, your punches results in a compromised defense.

An example of this can be illustrated with an uppercut as seen on the right. To properly throw an uppercut without compromising your defense, lower your forearm so that your elbow has between a 30- to 90-degree angle. Simultaneously, rotate around the waist to throw the uppercut upward and outward toward your target. If you wind your punch by pulling your elbow backward, rather than lowering your elbow, you will expose your chin, which compromises your defense.

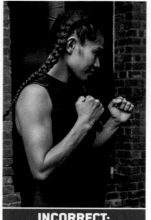

INCORRECT: GUARD TOO LOW

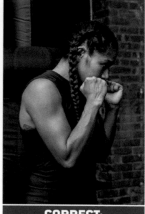

CORRECT: TIGHT GUARD

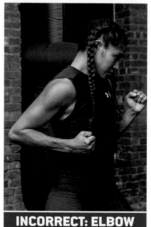

INCORRECT: ELBOW PULLED BACK

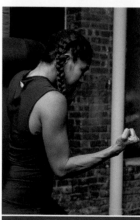

CORRECT: OPEN ELBOW

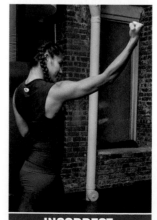

INCORRECT: OVEREXTENSION

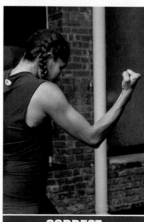

CORRECT EXTENSION

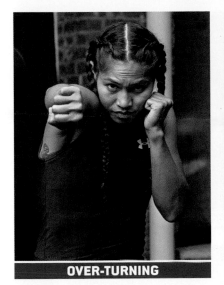

OVER-TURNING

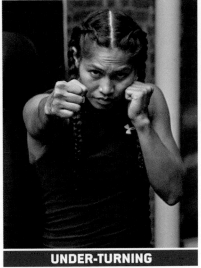

UNDER-TURNING

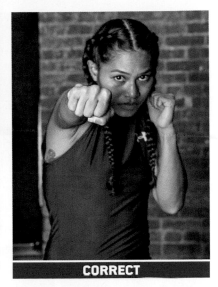

CORRECT

Over- and under-turning punches: In your neutral stance, your forearms should be parallel to each other. As you extend your arm out to throw straight punches (jab and cross), your wrist should be rotating so that upon full extension (without locking your arm), your knuckles are aligned horizontally. Over-turning or under-turning your punches results in directing force away from your target and may lessen the impact of your punch.

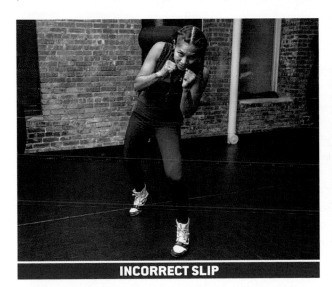

INCORRECT SLIP

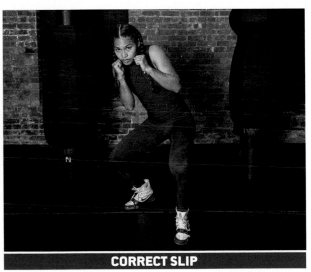

CORRECT SLIP

Shifting shoulders vs. slipping: Proper slipping entails moving your head off the center line of attack. Although alternating and shifting your shoulders forward mimics slipping, it does little to change your head position, which compromises your defense. In the incorrect image, the boxer shifts her shoulders forward, alternating sides through rotation around her waist. Notice her head position, which remains in the center line of attack. In the correct image, the boxer bends laterally around the waist from side to side to change her head position away from the center line of attack.

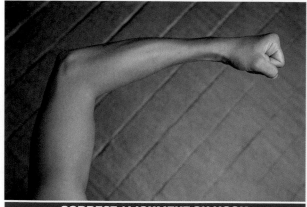

CORRECT ALIGNMENT ON HOOK

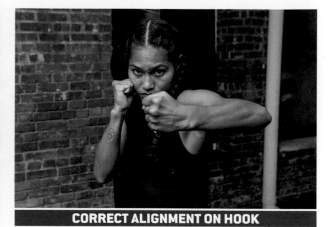

CORRECT ALIGNMENT ON HOOK

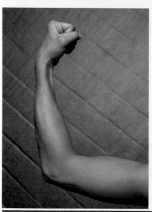
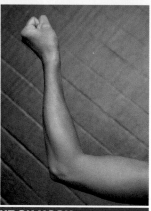

MISALIGNMENT ON HOOK

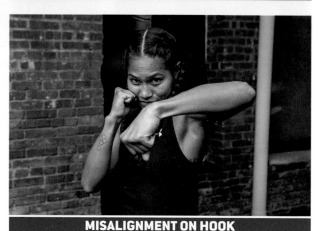

MISALIGNMENT ON HOOK

Three-point joint alignment: To avoid common elbow and wrist injuries, make sure that you have a three-point joint alignment when throwing punches. You generate a great amount of power when engaging your hips to throw punches, so you must ensure a proper support structure behind the knuckles and wrist, the joints that bear the brunt of the force generated by your hips.

When throwing straight punches (jab or cross), make sure that your wrists, elbows, and shoulders are aligned. Your wrists, elbows, and shoulders should be aligned for hooks to the head; knuckles, wrists, and elbows should be aligned for hooks to the body. Make sure that your knuckles, wrists, and elbows are aligned when throwing uppercuts.

SHADOWBOXING EXERCISES (ORTHODOX STANCE)

In this section, you will implement what you have learned so far. These exercises focus on repetition of certain punches and footwork, as well as calisthenics to develop muscle memory and coordination. You will need the following:

- Smartphone boxing timer set for 3-minute work rounds and 30-second rest periods
- A mirror, to view form and technique
- Boxing heavy bag (optional)

ROUND 1
Jab, cross, left hook.
Tips: Make sure you are turning your wrists on both the jab and cross to ensure you connect to the target with your knuckles. Lift your elbow and lock the joint to have an inner angle of 90 degrees as you rotate around the waist to throw the hook; make sure your wrist, elbow, and shoulder are aligned and level.

Slip side to side.
Tips: Make sure that your head is off the center line when you slip from one side to the other by bending laterally around the waist. Remember that when you slip in the direction adjacent to your rear foot, knees should point away from each other. When you slip in the direction adjacent to your lead foot, your knees should point forward.

Bounce.
Tips: Start by bouncing up and down on both feet. Then begin to transfer your entire body weight from one foot to the other.

Jab, cross, left hook, uppercut, left hook, cross.
Tips: Without pulling your elbow behind you, lower your rear forearm so the inner angle of your elbow is 45 degrees as you rotate around the waist to throw the rear uppercut. You may also alternate with the lead uppercut using the same mechanics.

Dip.
Tips: Make sure you take your hands with you as you level change; keep hands level with your chin.

Slip side to side.
Tips: Bend laterally around the waist from one side to the other as you keep your hands by your chin.

Pivot 90 degrees.
Tips: Lower your level slightly as you drive your rear foot into the floor, creating momentum to pivot on the ball of your lead foot.

Pivot back 90 degrees.
Tips: Drive your rear foot into the floor as you pivot on the ball of your lead foot to return to your initial position.

Last 30 seconds of round: pendulum steps (pages 27–30).

Tips: Remember to shift your weight over the foot on the center "X" by leaning your shoulders forward, backward, and from side to side.

ROUND 2
Cross, left hook, cross.

Tips: Make sure that you rotate around the waist as you extend your arm to throw the cross. Turn your wrist so that you connect on your knuckles. Lift your elbow and lock the joint to have an inner angle of 90 degrees. Make sure that the wrist, elbow, and shoulder are aligned and level when you throw the left hook.

Bounce.
Check hook, cross to the body, left uppercut, cross, jab.

Tips: When you throw the check hook, make sure that you pivot and throw the hook simultaneously. Lower your level by bending your knees as you throw the cross to the body. Plant your rear heel into the floor as you rotate around the waist to throw the lead uppercut.

Bounce.
Retreat and circle counter-clockwise.

Tips: Push off the lead foot to retreat and step backward, creating space between you and the target. Keep your feet parallel as you circle counter-clockwise. Make sure that whenever you stop circling, you are in your ready stance.

Bounce.
Slip side to side.
Bounce.
Cross, left hook, cross, left uppercut, cross, left hook.

Tips: Aim for speed with this combination. Avoid overextending the punches to improve speed.

Bounce.
Step to the left and pivot on lead foot.

Tips: Push off the rear foot. Your weight should be on your lead foot as you pivot.

Bounce.
Last 30 seconds of round: pendulum steps (pages 27–30).

ROUND 3
Jab, slip right, cross, jab, slip left, left hook.

Tips: Make sure to point your knees away from each other when slipping right. When slipping to the left, your knees should point forward, in the direction of your target.

Jab, dip, cross, left hook.

Tips: The aim of the dip is to rapidly lower your level to avoid incoming punches. Make sure that you quickly bend your knees to lower your level and catch your weight once you're in a squat position. Then extend your knees to ascend and return to your neutral stance.

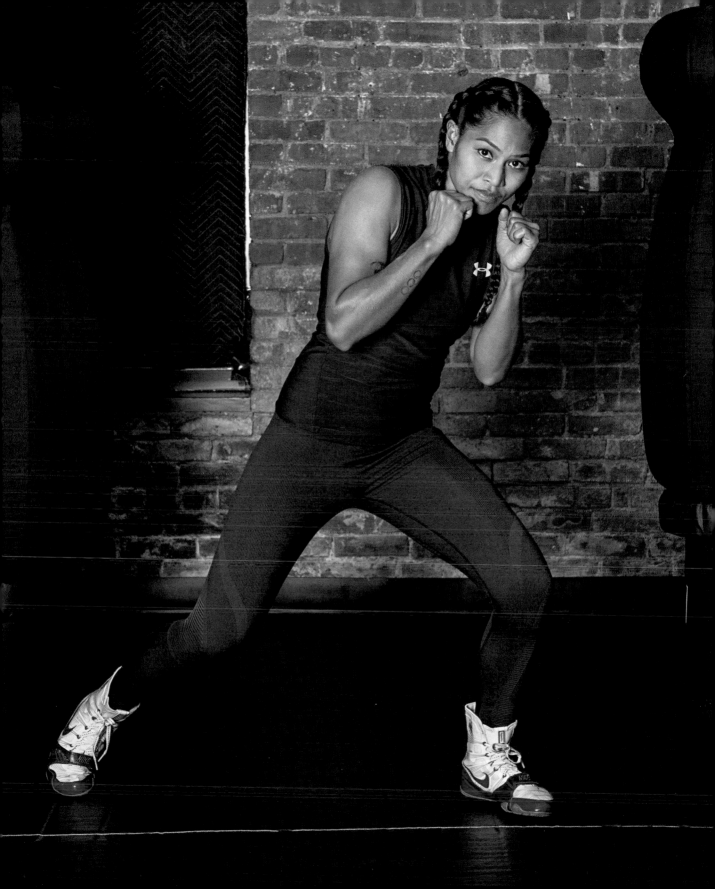

Jab, dip, left hook, cross.
Jab, catch with right elbow, right uppercut.

Tips: Remember that to catch, you should keep your fist by your chin and drop your shoulder so that your elbow lowers to your hip. Keep your elbow tucked in and pressed tight against your hip. Pivot on the rear foot as you throw the right uppercut.

Jab, catch with left elbow, left uppercut.

Tips: To catch, keep your fist by your chin and drop your left shoulder so that your elbow lowers to your hip. Keep your elbow tucked in and pressed tightly against your hip to absorb any impact.

Jab, catch with right elbow, right uppercut, left hook.
Jab, catch with left elbow, left uppercut, cross.

Tips: Extend your knees slightly when throwing the left uppercut, then slightly pivot on the ball of the rear foot so your toes are pointed forward when throwing the cross.

Jab, half step back, jab, cross, left uppercut.

Tips: Keep your lead foot in place as you take a half step back with the rear foot. You can lean your shoulders back slightly to create more distance between you and a punch that is closing in quickly.

Jab, slip right, right uppercut, left hook.
Jab, slip right, right uppercut, left hook, cross.
Last 30 seconds of round: pendulum steps (pages 27–30).

CALISTHENIC ROUND
1 minute Kick-Back Burpee to Plank Push-Ups (page 69).
1 minute Jump Squats (page 62).
1 minute Mountain Climber Burpees (page 70).

ROUND 4
Jab and step off right, step back with right uppercut.

Tips: Push off the right foot to bring your weight back to the center line in your boxing stance. Keep the lead foot in place.

Cross and step off left, step back with left hook.
Step back left uppercut, right uppercut.

Tips: Push off the lead foot to move your body backward. Bend your knees as you step backward, further lowering your level. Extend your knees slightly as you throw the left uppercut. Pivot on the ball of the rear foot as you throw the right uppercut.

Step forward right uppercut, left uppercut.

Tips: Push off the rear foot to move your body forward. Bend your knees as you step forward, lowering your level. Plant your rear heel into the floor as you throw the left uppercut.

Step forward left uppercut, cross, left hook.

Tips: Pivot on the ball of the rear foot as you throw the cross. Lift your left elbow up so that your wrist, elbow, and shoulder are aligned as you rotate around the waist to throw the left hook.

Step back right uppercut, left uppercut, left hook.

Tips: Throw the left uppercut and then lift your left elbow as you rotate around the waist to throw the left hook.

Last 30 seconds of round: pendulum steps (pages 27–30).

ROUND 5

Alternating jab, cross, left uppercut, cross, jab, right uppercut. Repeat this continuous punching sequence throughout the round.

Tips: Break the sequence into three-punch combinations: first jab, cross, left uppercut; then cross, jab, right uppercut. Aim to combine the two combinations into one continuous flow of nonstop punches. Make sure that you are using your reach on the straight punches (jab and cross) by extending your arms without locking your elbows.

ROUND 6

Cross, jab, cross, left uppercut, dip.

Tips: Advance first as you throw each punch. Then retreat as you throw the same punch combination. Maintain a lowered level throughout the exercise.

ROUND 7

Pendulum steps (pages 27–30).

Tips: Start the pendulum step exercise in one spot. For an added challenge, move around the available space while maintaining proper technique.

ROUND 8

Probe jab, right uppercut, cross, left uppercut.

Tips: The probe jab is an extended jab used as a measuring rod to maintain distance between you and your target, keeping you out of striking range. Hold your extended jab for 1 to 2 seconds and then throw a counter right uppercut, cross, and left uppercut.

CORE ROUND

50 Hand-to-Toe Crunches (page 74).
50 Elbow-to-Knee Crunches (page 75).
50 Pulse Crunches (page 75).

ROUND 9
Alternating jab, cross, left uppercut, cross, jab, right uppercut. Repeat this continuous punching sequence throughout the round.

Tips: Break the sequence into three-punch combinations: first jab, cross, left uppercut; then cross, jab, right uppercut. Aim to combine the two combinations into one continuous flow of nonstop punches. Make sure that you are using your reach on the straight punches (jab and cross) by extending your arms without locking your elbows.

ROUND 10
Left uppercut with lead foot step back, cross with rear foot step to angle off.

Tips: Throw the left uppercut as you step your lead foot backward, past the rear foot. Throw the cross as you pivot 90 degrees outward on the ball of your left foot and step your right foot backward to reset into neutral stance.

ROUND 11
Jab, cross, step forward with left uppercut, cross.

Tips: Step forward to switch to a right foot lead as you throw the lead uppercut. As you throw the cross, pivot 90 degrees inward on the ball of your right foot and step your left foot forward, past your right foot, to reset into neutral stance.

ROUND 12
Jab, step off with cross to the body, pendulum step, right uppercut, left hook, cross.

Tips: Step off to the left with the lead foot as you throw the cross to the target. After landing the cross, use the pendulum step so that you are facing the target's right lateral aspect. Follow up with the rear uppercut, left hook, and then cross.

SHADOWBOXING EXERCISES (SOUTHPAW STANCE)

In this section, you will implement what you have learned so far. These exercises focus on repetition of certain punches and footwork as well as calisthenics to develop muscle memory and coordination. You will need the following:

- Smartphone boxing timer set for 3-minute work rounds and 30-second rest periods

- A mirror, to view form and technique

- Boxing heavy bag (optional)

ROUND 1
Jab, cross, right hook.
Tips: Make sure you are turning your wrists on both the jab and cross to ensure you connect to the target with your knuckles. Lift your elbow and lock the joint to have an inner angle of 90 degrees as you rotate around the waist to throw the hook; make sure your wrist, elbow, and shoulder are aligned and level.

Slip side to side.
Tips: Make sure that your head is off the center line when you slip from one side to the other by bending laterally around the waist. Remember that when you slip in the direction adjacent to your rear foot, knees should point away from each other. When you slip in the direction adjacent to your lead foot, your knees should point forward.

Bounce.
Tips: Start by bouncing up and down on both feet. Make sure that you are transferring your entire body weight from one foot to the other.

Jab, cross, right hook, left uppercut, right hook, cross.
Tips: Without pulling your elbow behind you, lower your rear forearm so the inner angle of your elbow is 45 degrees as you rotate around the waist to throw the rear uppercut. You may also alternate with the lead uppercut using the same mechanics.

Dip.
Tips: Make sure you take your hands with you as you level change; keep hands level with your chin.

Slip side to side.
Tips: Bend laterally around the waist from one side to the other as you keep your hands by your chin.

Pivot 90 degrees.
Tips: Lower your level slightly as you drive your rear foot into the floor, creating momentum to pivot on the ball of your lead foot.

Pivot back 90 degrees.
Tips: Drive your rear foot into the floor as you pivot on the ball of your lead foot to return to your initial position.

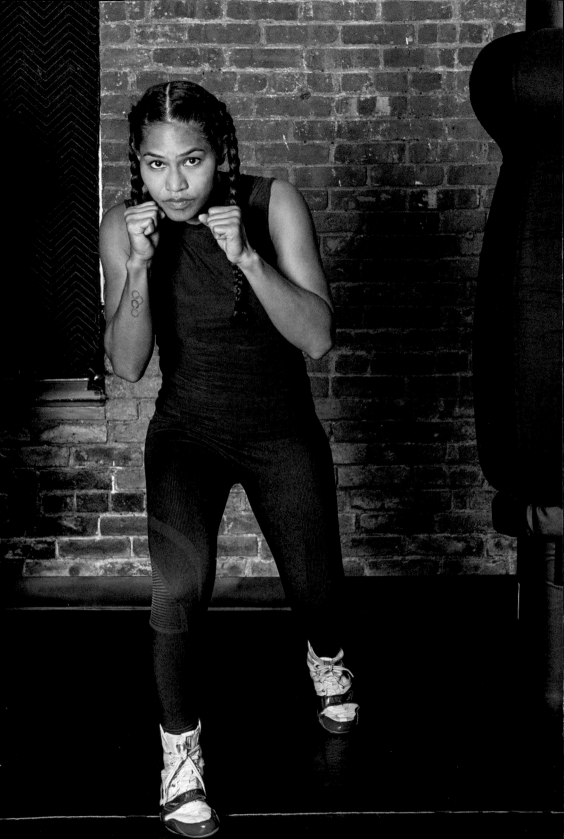

Last 30 seconds of round: pendulum steps (pages 27–30).

Tips: Remember to shift your weight over the foot on the center "X" by leaning your shoulders forward, backward, and from side to side.

ROUND 2
Cross, right hook, cross.

Tips: Make sure that you rotate around the waist as you extend your arm to throw the cross. Turn your wrist so that you connect on your knuckles. Lift your elbow and lock the joint to have an inner angle of 90 degrees. Make sure that the wrist, elbow, and shoulder are aligned and level when you throw the right hook.

Bounce.
Check hook, cross to the body, lead uppercut, cross, jab.

Tips: When you throw the check hook, make sure that you pivot and throw the hook simultaneously. Lower your level by bending your knees as you throw the cross to the body. Plant your rear heel into the floor as you rotate around the waist to throw the lead uppercut.

Bounce.
Retreat and circle counter-clockwise.

Tips: Push off the lead foot to retreat and step backward, creating space between you and the target. Keep your feet parallel as you circle counter-clockwise. Make sure that whenever you stop circling, you are in your ready stance.

Bounce.
Slip side to side.
Bounce.
Cross, right hook, cross, right uppercut, cross, right hook.

Tips: Aim for speed with this combination. Avoid overextending the punches to improve speed.

Bounce.
Step to the left and pivot on lead foot.

Tips: Push off the rear foot. Your weight should be on your lead foot as you pivot.

Bounce.
Last 30 seconds of round: pendulum steps (pages 27–30).

ROUND 3
Jab, slip left, cross, jab, slip right, right hook.

Tips: Make sure to point your knees away from each other when slipping left. When slipping to the right, your knees should point forward, in the direction of your target.

Jab, dip, cross, lead right hook.

Tips: The aim of the dip is to rapidly lower your level to avoid incoming punches. Make sure that you quickly bend your knees to lower your level and catch your weight once you're in a squat position. Then extend your knees to ascend and return to your neutral stance.

Jab, dip, lead hook, cross.
Jab, catch with left elbow, left uppercut.

Tips: Remember that to catch, you should keep your fist by your chin and drop your shoulder so that your elbow lowers to your hip. Keep your elbow tucked in and pressed tight against your hip. Pivot on the rear foot as you throw the left uppercut.

Jab, catch with right elbow, right uppercut.

Tips: To catch, keep your fist by your chin and drop your right shoulder so that your elbow lowers to your hip. Keep your elbow tucked in and pressed tightly against your hip to absorb any impact.

Jab, catch with left elbow, left uppercut, right hook.
Jab, catch with right elbow, right uppercut, cross.

Tips: Extend your knees slightly when throwing the right uppercut, then slightly pivot on the ball of the rear foot so your toes are pointed forward when throwing the cross.

Jab, half step back, jab, cross, right uppercut.

Tips: Keep your lead foot in place as you take a half step back with the rear foot. You can lean your shoulders back slightly to create more distance between you and a punch that is closing in quickly.

Jab, slip left, left uppercut, right hook.
Jab, slip left, left uppercut, right hook, cross.
Last 30 seconds of round: pendulum steps (pages 27–30).

CALISTHENIC ROUND
1 minute Kick-Back Burpee to Plank Push-Ups (page 69).
1 minute Jump Squats (page 62).
1 minute Mountain Climber Burpees (page 70).

ROUND 4
Jab and step off left, step back with left uppercut.

Tips: Push off the left foot to bring your weight back to the center line in your boxing stance. Keep the lead foot in place.

Cross and step off right, step back with right hook.
Step back right uppercut, left uppercut.

Tips: Push off the lead foot to move your body backward. Bend your knees as you step backward, further lowering your level. Extend your knees slightly as you throw the right uppercut. Pivot on the ball of the rear foot as you throw the left uppercut.

Step forward left uppercut, right uppercut.

Tips: Push off the rear foot to move your body forward. Bend your knees as you step forward, lowering your level. Plant your rear heel into the floor as you throw the right uppercut.

Step forward right uppercut, cross, right hook.

Tips: Pivot on the ball of the rear foot as you throw the cross. Lift your right elbow up so that your wrist, elbow, and shoulder are aligned as you rotate around the waist to throw the right hook.

Step back left uppercut, right uppercut, right hook.

Tips: Throw the right uppercut and then lift your left elbow as you rotate around the waist to throw the right hook.

Last 30 seconds of round: pendulum steps (pages 27–30).

ROUND 5

Alternating jab, cross, right uppercut, cross, jab, left uppercut. Repeat this continuous punching sequence throughout the round.

Tips: Break the sequence into three-punch combinations: first jab, cross, right uppercut; then cross, jab, left uppercut. Aim to combine the two combinations into one continuous flow of nonstop punches. Make sure that you are using your reach on the straight punches (jab and cross) by extending your arms without locking your elbows.

ROUND 6

Cross, jab, cross, right uppercut, dip.

Tips: Advance first as you throw each punch. Then retreat as you throw the same punch combination. Maintain a lowered level throughout the exercise.

ROUND 7

Pendulum steps (pages 27–30).

Tips: Start the pendulum step exercise in one spot. For an added challenge, move around the available space while maintaining proper technique.

ROUND 8

Probe jab, left uppercut, cross, right uppercut.

Tips: The probe jab is an extended jab used as a measuring rod to maintain distance between you and your target, keeping you out of striking range. Hold your extended jab for 1 to 2 seconds and then throw a counter left uppercut, cross, and right uppercut.

CORE ROUND

50 Hand-to-Toe Crunches (page 74).
50 Elbow-to-Knee Crunches (page 75).
50 Pulse Crunches (page 75).

ROUND 9

Alternating jab, cross, right uppercut, cross, jab, left uppercut. Repeat this continuous punching sequence throughout the round.

Tips: Break the sequence into three-punch combinations: first jab, cross, right uppercut; then cross, jab, left uppercut. Aim to combine the two combinations into one continuous flow of nonstop punches. Make sure that you are using your reach on the straight punches (jab and cross) by extending your arms without locking your elbows.

ROUND 10

Right uppercut with lead foot step back, cross with rear foot step to angle off.

Tips: Throw the right uppercut as you step your lead foot backward, past the rear foot. Throw the cross as you pivot 90 degrees outward on the ball of your right foot and step your left foot backward to reset into neutral stance.

ROUND 11

Jab, cross, step forward with lead uppercut, cross.

Tips: Step forward to switch to a left foot lead as you throw the lead uppercut. As you throw the cross, pivot 90 degrees inward on the ball of your left foot and step your right foot forward, past your left foot, to reset into neutral stance.

ROUND 12

Jab, step off with cross to the body, pendulum step, left uppercut, right hook, cross.

Tips: Step off to the right with the lead foot as you throw the cross to the target. After landing the cross, use the pendulum step so that you are facing the target's left lateral aspect. Follow up with the left uppercut, right hook, and then cross.

CHAPTER 5

BOXING ROUNDS

In this chapter, you will incorporate plyometric and core exercises along with shadowboxing. Improving endurance as you employ proper mechanics helps your body reinforce muscle memory. Additionally, improved endurance allows you to maintain your defense, since fatigue may cause you to lower your guard (dropping your hands and/or flaring your elbows), which would compromise your form and ability to defend against counterpunches.

ORTHODOX STANCE

You will need the following:

- Smartphone boxing timer set for 3-minute work rounds and 30-second rest periods
- A mirror, to view form and technique
- Boxing heavy bag (optional)

ROUND 1

Jab, cross, diagonal step throwing left hook, cross.

Tips: Make sure to keep your elbows tucked in to avoid telegraphing your punches. Turn your wrists as you throw the jab and cross to connect on the knuckles of your fist. Remember to extend your arms without locking your elbow. Take a diagonal step forward with your right foot so that it is slightly ahead of your left foot as you throw the left hook. Pivot on the ball of your right foot as you throw the cross.

ROUND 2

Jab, cross, diagonal step throwing left uppercut, cross.

Tips: Take a diagonal step forward with your right foot so that it is slightly ahead of your left foot as you throw the left uppercut. Pivot on the ball of your right foot as you throw the cross.

PLYOMETRIC ROUND
Jumping Lunges (page 68): 3 sets.
Jump Squats (page 62): 3 sets.

ROUND 3
Jab, cross, step right throwing left hook to the body, cross.

ROUND 4
Level change, jab to your target's head, then jab to your target's body and quickly follow up with a cross, step to the right as you weave to avoid any counterpunches, continue to circle out.

Tips: Keep your hands by your chin as you level change. Keep your lead arm extended as you circle out and away from any potential advance and counter.

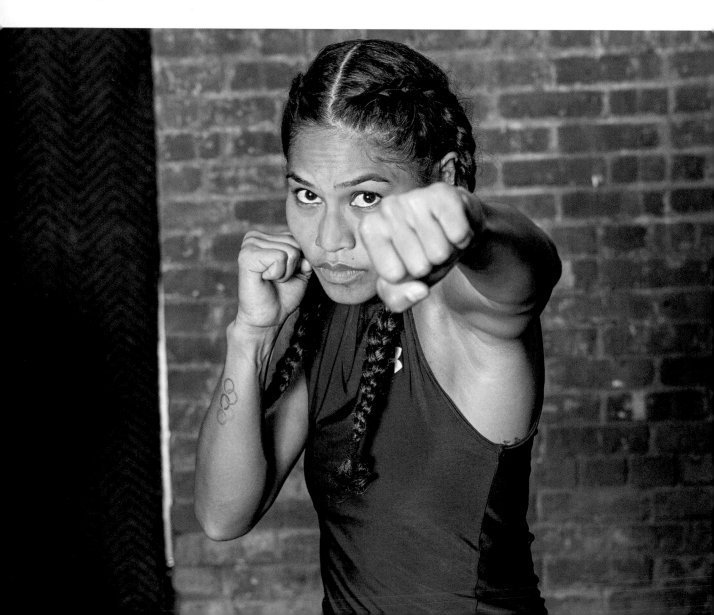

CORE ROUND
360-Degree Abs (page 76).

ROUND 5
Jab, up-jab, left hook, step left, pivot on lead foot, continue to circle left.

Tips: Turn your wrist on the jab to connect your knuckles to the target. Retract and lower your left forearm so that your fist is level to your naval, locking your elbow at an angle slightly wider than 90 degrees. Without decreasing the inner angle of your elbow, use your shoulder to lever the upward motion on the up-jab. Retract. Lift and lock your left elbow at 90 degrees and rotate around the waist to throw the left hook.

ROUND 6
Nonstop jab and cross.

Tips: Start in your neutral boxing stance with your hands by your chin. Turn your wrists when throwing the jab and cross. Make sure that you are fully extending your arms without locking your elbows. Make sure that on the retraction of each punch, you are returning your hands to your chin and not lowering them down to your chest, which compromises your defense. Focus on maintaining proper punching technique and keeping a strong defense throughout this round.

PLYOMETRIC ROUND
Jumping Lunges (page 68): 3 sets.
Jump Squats (page 62): 3 sets.

ROUND 7
Up-jab, cross, left hook to the body, left hook to the head.

Tips: When throwing the left hook to the body, slip slightly to the left as you lower your left forearm (without pulling your elbow back) so that the inner angle of your elbow is 90-degrees. Rotate around the waist to connect with the knuckles of your fist.

ROUND 8
Jab, cross, left hook to the head, left hook to the body, pivot.

Tips: To throw the left hook to the head, lift and lock your left elbow at 90 degrees as you rotate around the waist. Retract. For the left hook to the body, slightly slip to the left as you drop your left hand, making a 90-degree angle in your elbow and then rotating around the waist. Lower your level slightly as you push off the rear foot and pivot on the ball of your lead foot 90 degrees.

SOUTHPAW STANCE

You will need the following:

- Smartphone boxing timer set for 3-minute work rounds and 30-second rest periods
- A mirror, to view form and technique
- Boxing heavy bag (optional)

ROUND 1

Jab, cross, diagonal step throwing right hook, cross.

Tips: Make sure to keep your elbows tucked in to avoid telegraphing your punches. Turn your wrists as you throw the jab and cross to connect on the knuckles of your fist. Remember to extend your arms without locking your elbow. Take a diagonal step forward with your left foot so that it is slightly ahead of your right foot as you throw the right hook. Pivot on the ball of your left foot as you throw the cross.

ROUND 2

Jab, cross, diagonal step throwing right uppercut, cross.

Tips: Take a diagonal step forward with your left foot so that it is slightly ahead of your right foot as you throw the right uppercut. Pivot on the ball of your left foot as you throw the cross.

PLYOMETRIC ROUND

Jumping Lunges (page 68): 3 sets.
Jump Squats (page 62): 3 sets.

ROUND 3

Jab, cross, step left throwing right hook to the body, cross.

ROUND 4

Level change, jab to your target's head, then jab to your target's body and quickly follow up with a cross, step to the left as you weave to avoid any counterpunches, continue to circle out.

Tips: Keep your hands by your chin as you level change. Keep your lead arm extended as you circle out and away from any potential advance and counter.

CORE ROUND

360-Degree Abs (page 76).

ROUND 5

Jab, up-jab, right hook, step right, pivot on lead foot, continue to circle right.

Tips: Turn your wrist on the jab to connect your knuckles to the target. Retract and lower your right forearm so that your fist is level to your naval, locking your elbow at an angle slightly wider than 90 degrees. Without decreasing the inner angle of your elbow, use your shoulder to lever the upward motion on the up-jab. Retract. Lift and lock your left elbow at 90 degrees and rotate around the waist to throw the right hook.

ROUND 6
Nonstop jab and cross.

Tips: Start in your neutral boxing stance with your hands by your chin. Turn your wrists when throwing the jab and cross. Make sure that you are fully extending your arms without locking your elbows. Make sure that on the retraction of each punch, you are returning your hands to your chin and not lowering them down to your chest, which compromises your defense. Focus on maintaining proper punching technique and keeping a strong defense throughout this round.

PLYOMETRIC ROUND
Jumping Lunges (page 68): 3 sets.
Jump Squats (page 62): 3 sets.

ROUND 7
Up-jab, cross, right hook to the body, right hook to the head.

Tips: When throwing the right hook to the body, slip slightly to the right as you lower your right forearm (without pulling your elbow back) so that the inner angle of your elbow is 90-degrees. Rotate around the waist to connect with the knuckles of your fist.

ROUND 8
Jab, cross, right hook to the head, right hook to the body, pivot.

Tips: To throw the right hook to the head, lift and lock your left elbow at 90 degrees as you rotate around the waist. Retract. For the right hook to the body, slightly slip to the right as you drop your right hand, making a 90-degree angle in your elbow and then rotating around the waist. Lower your level slightly as you push off the rear foot and pivot on the ball of your lead foot 90 degrees.

BOXING CIRCUIT

This chapter provides you with circuits so you can vary intensity and switch up exercises in your training regimen. The circuits incorporate exercises that aim to improve both cardiovascular endurance as well as technique.

CIRCUIT I

When you are doing exercises from Station II, focus on technique and maintaining a strong defense after every punch. This means keep your hands up to protect your chin, tuck your elbows in to protect your body, use your reach and turn your wrists to connect your knuckles to the target, and retract your hands back to your chin after throwing every punch. Avoid crowding your punches when you get to the exercises on Station IV by keeping a measured distance between your body and the heavy bag. You will also be doing some plyometric exercises in Stations I and III to build overall endurance.

What you will need:

- Smartphone interval timer set to 3-2-1-1-2-minute work periods and 15-second rest periods at each station
- Jump rope
- 2-pound dumbbells
- Velcro boxing gloves
- Boxing heavy bag
- Mirror to view form and technique (optional)

Warm-Up
Jump rope for 8 minutes

Station I (3 minutes)
- Interval I: Jump Rope (page 64)
- Interval II: Double-Under Jump (page 64)
- Interval III: Jump Rope
- Interval IV: Double-Under Jump

Station II (2 minutes)

- Interval I: Nonstop jab and cross with 2-pound weights

- Interval II: Nonstop jab, cross, left uppercut, cross, jab, right uppercut with 2-pound weights (Southpaw: Nonstop jab, cross, right uppercut, cross, jab, left uppercut with 2-pound weights)

- Interval III: Nonstop jab and cross with 2-pound weights

- Interval IV: Nonstop jab, cross, left uppercut, cross, jab, right uppercut with 2-pound weights (Southpaw: Nonstop jab, cross, right uppercut, cross, jab, left uppercut with 2-pound weights)

Station III (1 minute)

- Interval I: Quick Feet to Sprawl (page 67)

- Interval II: 4 Mountain Climber Burpees (page 70)

- Interval III: Quick Feet to Sprawl

- Interval IV: 4 Mountain Climber Burpees

Break to put gloves on (1 minute)

Station IV: Heavy bag (2 minutes)

- Interval I: Cross, left hook (right for southpaw), cross, double jab. Repeat combination every 2 to 3 seconds with minimal rest in between.

- Interval II: Jab, cross, left hook to the head, left hook to the body, pivot out, cross, left hook to the head, cross. (Southpaw: Jab, cross, right hook to the head, right hook to the body, pivot out, cross, right hook to the head, cross.) Repeat combination every 2 to 3 seconds with minimal rest in between.

- Interval III: Cross, left hook, cross, double jab. (Southpaw: Cross, right hook, cross, double jab.) Repeat combination every 2 to 3 seconds with minimal rest in between.

- Interval IV: Jab, cross, left hook to the head, left hook to the body, pivot out, cross, left hook to the head, cross. (Southpaw: Jab, cross, right hook to the head, right hook to the body, pivot out, cross, right hook to the head, cross.) Repeat combination every 2 to 3 seconds with minimal rest in between.

CIRCUIT II

When you are doing exercises from Station I focus on speed, technique, and maintaining a strong defense after every punch. This means keep your hands up to protect your chin, tuck your elbows in to protect your body, use your reach and turn your wrists to connect your knuckles to the target, and retract your hands back to your chin after throwing every punch. Exercises from Station II will focus more on power, technique, and maintaining a strong defense after every punch. Make sure that as you alternate sides when throwing the body shots (hooks) that you always have one hand protecting your chin while the other hand delivers the punch. Additionally, sit on your punches, rotate around the waist, and pivot on the rear foot to allow your hips to generate power. You will also be doing some plyometric exercises in Station III as well as several variations of push-ups in Station IV to build overall endurance.

What you will need:

- Smartphone interval timer set for 1-minute work rounds and 15-second rest periods at each station
- Velcro boxing gloves
- Boxing heavy bag

- Step-up block
- Jump rope
- Optional: Yoga mat

Warm-Up
Jump rope for 8 minutes

Station I: Heavy bag, continuous punching (1 minute per interval)

- Interval I: jab and cross
- Interval II: hooks
- Interval III: uppercuts
- Interval IV: jab and cross
- Interval V: hooks
- Interval VI: uppercuts

Station II: Heavy bag (1 minute per interval)

- Interval I through Interval VI: Nonstop body shots with power

Station III (1 minute per interval)

- Interval I: Jump Squats (page 62) (max repetitions)
- Interval II: Wall sit (lean your back against the wall, descend into a 90-degree squat, and hold position)
- Interval III: 4 repetitions knee-to-elbow mountain climber then 1 repetition burpee (page 70 without step 2)
- Interval IV: Jump Squats (max repetitions)
- Interval V: Wall sit
- Interval VI: 4 repetitions knee-to-elbow mountain climber then 1 repetition burpee (page 70 without step 2)

Station IV (1 minute per interval)

- Interval I: Push-Ups (page 58) (max repetitions)

- Interval II: Jump Squats (page 62) (max repetitions)

- Interval III: Push-Ups (max repetitions)

- Interval IV: Push-Ups (max repetitions)

- Interval V: Jump Squats (max repetitions)

- Interval VI: Push-Ups (max repetitions)

CIRCUIT III

This endurance circuit is designed to give you a full-body workout. Refer to the Muscular Endurance section in Chapter 4 to switch up endurance exercises for this circuit. Rather than using a timer for this circuit, complete the recommended amount of repetitions for each exercise.

What you will need:

- BOSU ball

- Pull-up bar

- Landmine

Station I
- BOSU Ball Jump Squats (page 63)

Station II
- Single-Arm Push Press with Landmine (page 56)

Station III
- Chin-Up to Pull-Up (page 61)

Station IV
- Thruster with Landmine (page 53)

This chapter includes over 50 punch combinations that you can incorporate when shadowboxing. Remember to pay close attention to your footwork and technique as you practice. Refer to previous chapters for more information on mechanics and specific movements. Remember to retract your hands after each punch.

COMBINATION 1
Jab, cross, hook

Turn your wrists on the jab and cross to connect your knuckles to the target. Rotate around the waist to shift your rear shoulder forward as you extend your rear arm and pivot on the ball of the rear foot to throw the cross. Your feet should be parallel to each other, pointing toward the target. Lift and lock your lead elbow at about 90 degrees, then rotate around the waist, squaring your hips toward the target, to throw the hook.

COMBINATION 2
Cross, hook, cross

To throw the hook, lift and lock your lead elbow at about 90 degrees, then rotate around the waist, squaring your hips toward the target. Remember not to over-rotate, as this will decrease the impact of your punch.

COMBINATION 3
Hook, cross, jab

Lift and lock lead elbow at about 90 degrees, then rotate around the waist to throw the hook. Remember to turn your wrists on the cross and jab to connect your knuckles to the target.

COMBINATION 4
Double jab, cross

Fully extend your arm (without locking elbow) to throw the jab, and then retract your arm halfway before throwing the second jab.

COMBINATION 5
Jab, double cross

Rotate around the waist to shift your rear shoulder forward and pivot on the ball of the rear foot to throw the second cross.

COMBINATION 6
Up-jab, cross, body shot

To throw the up-jab, lower your lead forearm so that your fist is level to your naval, locking the inner angle of your elbow at 90 degrees. Then, without decreasing the inner angle of your elbow, use your shoulder to lever the upward motion on the up-jab. To throw the body shot, drop your lead hand to get a 45-degree angle in your elbow joint and rotate around the waist. Remember not to over-rotate.

COMBINATION 7
Body shot, hook, cross

Lower your lead forearm until the inner angle of your elbow is 90 degrees and rotate around the waist to throw the body shot with the lead hand. Then, lift and lock your lead elbow at about 90 degrees and rotate around the waist to throw the hook.

COMBINATION 8
Jab, double body shot

To throw a double body shot, lower your rear forearm to get a 90-degree angle in your elbow, rotate around the waist, and pivot on the ball of your rear foot as you connect the body shot with the knuckles on your fist. Retract and repeat with your lead hand. Plant your rear heel into the ground as throw the body shot with your lead hand (do not pivot your lead foot).

COMBINATION 9
Jab, body shot with rear hand, thrust with lead hand

After you throw your body shot, throw the thrust punch by lowering your lead forearm to get a 90-degree inner angle in your elbow, then rotate around the waist and connect the knuckles of your fist to the center line of the body of your target.

COMBINATION 10
Uppercut, hook, cross

Make sure that your wrist, elbow, and shoulder are parallel when throwing the hook.

COMBINATION 11
Jab, uppercut, cross

Do not pull your elbow back to start throwing the uppercut, as doing so exposes your chin to make you an open target.

COMBINATION 12
Step off, hook, cross

Take a lateral step with the rear foot, keeping the lead foot in place, as you lift your elbow. Simultaneously, rotate around the waist to throw the lead hook. Step the rear foot back to its initial position as you turn your wrist and extend your rear arm to throw the cross.

COMBINATION 13
Step off, cross, hook
Take a lateral step with the lead foot, keeping the rear foot in place, as you turn your wrist and extend your rear arm to throw the cross. Step the lead foot back to its initial position as you lift your elbow. Simultaneously, rotate around the waist to throw the lead hook. Make sure that your wrist, elbow, and shoulder are parallel when you throw the hook.

COMBINATION 14
Step off, jab, rear uppercut
Take a lateral step with the rear foot, keeping the lead foot in place, as you turn your wrist and extend your lead arm to throw the jab. Step the rear foot back to its initial position as you throw the rear uppercut.

COMBINATION 15
Step off, double jab
Take a forward step with the lead foot, keeping the rear foot in place, as you turn your wrist and extend your lead arm to throw the jab. Lower your level as you throw a second jab to the body of the target.

COMBINATION 16
Jab, cross, jab
Turn your wrist on the jab and cross to connect your knuckles to the target. Retract after each punch.

COMBINATION 17
Jab, cross, lead uppercut
Turn your wrist on the jab and cross to connect your knuckles to the target. When throwing the lead uppercut, make sure to lower your lead forearm (try not to pull your elbow behind you) and rotate around the waist.

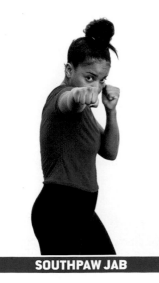

SOUTHPAW JAB

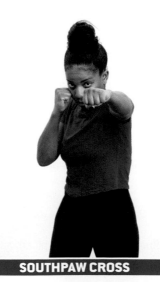

SOUTHPAW CROSS

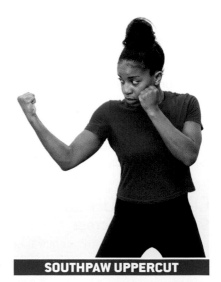

SOUTHPAW UPPERCUT

COMBINATION 18
Cross, body shot, hook

Pivot on your rear foot, rotate around the waist, and extend your arm to throw the cross and add reach to your punch. Unwind at the waist and plant your rear heel into the ground as you throw the body shot.

COMBINATION 19
Cross, lead uppercut, cross

Remember to rotate around the waist, shift you rear shoulder forward, and pivot on the ball of the rear foot to throw the cross. For the uppercut, drop your forearm to get between a 45 and 90-degree angle in your elbow, then rotate around the waist to throw the punch upward and outward.

COMBINATION 20
Cross, uppercut, cross, hook

After throwing the second cross, lift and lock your lead elbow at 90 degrees and rotate around the waist to throw the hook.

COMBINATION 21
Cross, uppercut, cross, hook, uppercut

After throwing the hook, starting with your elbow in front and by your waist, drop your hand to get between a 45 and 90-degree angle in your elbow, and rotate around the waist to throw the uppercut upward and outward.

COMBINATION 22
Jab, lead hook, cross

After retracting the jab, lift and lock your lead elbow at 90 degrees and rotate around the waist to throw the hook. Retract and throw the cross.

COMBINATION 23
Cross, hook, slip, uppercut, cross

Throw the cross, then lift and lock your elbow at an inner angle of 90 degrees as you rotate around the waist to throw the lead hook. Slip slightly by bending laterally around the waist as you lower your lead forearm until you have about a 45-degree inner angle in your elbow, and rotate around the waist as you throw the lead uppercut upward and outward. Throw a second cross.

COMBINATION 24
Jab, up-jab, cross

To throw the up-jab, lower your lead forearm so that your fist is level to your naval, locking the inner angle of your elbow at 90-degrees. Then, use your shoulder to lever the upward motion on the up-jab. Rotate around the waist to shift your rear shoulder forward as you extend your rear arm, and pivot on the ball of your rear foot to throw the cross.

COMBINATION 25
Jab, hook, jab
To throw the hook, lift and lock your lead elbow at 90 degrees and rotate around the waist. Retract halfway then throw the second jab.

COMBINATION 26
Jab, double lead hook
To throw the hook, lift and lock your lead elbow at 90 degrees and rotate around the waist. Keep your elbow lifted, move your arm in a circular motion, and rotate at the waist to throw the second hook. Retract.

COMBINATION 27
Hook, cross, hook
Lift and lock your lead elbow at 90 degrees and rotate around the waist to throw the hook. Rotate around the waist to shift your rear shoulder forward, extend your rear arm, and pivot on the ball of the rear foot to throw the cross.

COMBINATION 28
Cross, weave, hook
After throwing the cross, weave by taking a lateral step with your rear foot as you lower your level and rotate around the waist. As you come back up, continue to rotate, lift and lock your lead elbow at 90 degrees, and throw the hook.

COMBINATION 29
Cross, step, check hook
After throwing the cross, take a short diagonal step forward and then pivot on your lead foot. At the same time, lift and lock your lead elbow at 90 degrees to throw the lead check hook as you pivot on the ball of your lead foot.

COMBINATION 30
Cross, step, jab, cross
After you throw the cross, take a short diagonal step forward with your lead foot and pivot on the ball of your lead foot. After you throw the jab, rotate around the waist to shift your rear shoulder forward and throw the cross. Retract.

COMBINATION 31
Jab, slip, cross
After you throw the jab, bend laterally around the waist to slip and move head off the center line. As you return to neutral stance, rotate around the waist to shift your rear shoulder forward and throw the cross.

COMBINATION 32
Jab, overhand, body shot, uppercut

After you throw the jab, weave forward and diagonally with your lead foot as you extend your rear arm in a circular motion, hitting the target in a downward motion. Rotate around the waist, lock your lead elbow in a 90-degree angle, and deliver the body shot. Make sure to protect your chin with your rear hand as you lower your lead forearm and rotate around the waist to throw the lead uppercut.

COMBINATION 33
Jab, overhand, body shot, uppercut, cross

Make sure to turn your wrists on the jab and cross to ensure you connect to the target with the knuckles of your fist. Throw the body shot with your lead hand. Throw the uppercut with your lead hand.

COMBINATION 34
Jab, slip, pivot, hook to body

After throwing the jab, bend laterally around the waist to take your head off the center line. Push off your rear foot and pivot on the ball of the lead foot to change direction 90 degrees. Take a slight lateral step with your lead foot as you rotate around the waist, locking your elbow at an inner angle of 90 degrees to throw the hook to the body with your rear hand. Retract.

COMBINATION 35
Jab, slip, body shot, hook

To slip, bend laterally around the waist to the side adjacent to your rear hand, taking your head off the center line. When throwing the body shot, use your rear hand and pivot your rear foot until your toes point forward. Your rear and lead foot should both face the target.

COMBINATION 36
Jab, slip, body shot, uppercut

Remember not to pull your elbow before throwing the uppercut, as this will expose the chin.

COMBINATION 37
Jab, slip, body shot, uppercut, cross

Remember to turn your wrist on the jab and the cross to connect your knuckles to the target.

COMBINATION 38
Jab, rear hook

While retracting from the jab, lift and lock your rear elbow at an inner angle of 90 degrees as you rotate around the waist to throw the hook. Pivot on the ball of the rear foot so your toes face forward when throwing the rear hook.

COMBINATION 39
Slip, lean back, slip

Bend laterally around the waist to the side adjacent to your rear hand, taking your head off the center line. Stay low as you lean back. Bend laterally around the waist in the opposite direction as you return to neutral, taking your head off the center line once again.

COMBINATION 40
Slip, lean back, slip, pivot

Bend laterally around the waist to the side adjacent to your rear hand. Stay low as you lean back. Bend laterally around the waist in the opposite direction. Push off your rear foot and pivot 90 degrees on the ball of your lead foot.

COMBINATION 41
Catch, cross, hook, cross

Start in neutral stance with your rear hand protecting your chin and elbow tucked against your side. Lift your rear shoulder up toward your ear to catch an incoming strike. Counter with a straight cross. Lift and lock your lead elbow at an inner angle of 90 degrees and rotate around the waist to throw the hook, then pivot on the ball of your rear foot while rotating your waist to throw a second cross.

COMBINATION 42
Catch, hook, cross

Start in neutral stance with your rear hand protecting your chin and elbow tucked against your side. Lift your lead shoulder up toward your ear to catch an incoming strike. Counter with a lead hook, then throw a cross.

COMBINATION 43
Catch, uppercut, hook, cross

Protect your chin with your rear hand, tuck your elbow against your side, and bend laterally around the waist to lower your elbow to your hip to catch an incoming strike. Counter with a rear uppercut by lowering your rear forearm and rotating at the waist to throw the punch upward and outward. Lift and lock your lead elbow at 90 degrees while rotating at the waist to throw the lead hook. Shift your rear shoulder forward as you extend your rear arm and pivot on the ball of the rear foot to throw the cross.

COMBINATION 44
Catch, uppercut, cross, hook

Protect your chin with your rear hand, tuck your elbow against your side, and bend laterally around the waist to lower your lead elbow to your hip to catch an incoming strike. Counter with a lead uppercut, cross, and lead hook.

COMBINATION 45
Parry, cross, jab

Turn the wrist of your rear hand so that your palm is facing your target and flick your wrist downward to deflect incoming straight punches. Quickly counter with a straight cross by extending your rear arm, rotating at the waist, and pivoting on the ball of your rear foot to add reach to your punch. Make sure to turn your wrist on the cross to connect on the knuckles of your fist. Retract. Throw the jab.

COMBINATION 46
Parry, jab

Parry, then quickly counter with a jab by turning your wrist as you extend your lead arm to connect your knuckles to the target.

COMBINATION 47
Jab, rear hook, body shot

After retracting your jab, lift and lock your rear elbow at an inner angle of 90 degrees while rotating at the waist to throw the rear hook. Lower your lead forearm so that the inner angle of your elbow is between 45 and 90 degrees as you rotate around the waist to throw the body shot with the lead hand.

COMBINATION 48
Jab, cross, slip, cross, hook

Turn your wrist on the jab and the cross to connect your knuckles to the target. Bend laterally around the waist to the side adjacent to your rear hand, taking your head off the center line. Return to neutral stance as you throw the second cross. Lift and lock your lead elbow at 90 degrees and rotate around the waist to throw the lead hook.

COMBINATION 49
Jab, up-jab, hook

To throw the up-jab, lower your lead forearm so that your fist is level to your naval, locking the inner angle of your elbow at 90 degrees. Then, without decreasing the inner angle of your elbow, use your shoulder to lever the upward motion on the up-jab. Follow up with the lead hook.

COMBINATION 50
Jab, cross, hook, pivot

Turn your wrist on the jab and the cross to connect your knuckles to the target. After throwing the lead hook, lower your level slightly by bending your knees. Then push off the rear foot and pivot on the ball of your lead foot 90 degrees.

COMBINATION 51
Alternating body shots, cross, hook
Lower your level slightly as you advance, closing distance to the target. Lower your rear forearm so that the inner angle of your elbow is 90 degrees. Drive your rear hand forward, thrusting the punch to the center line of the target; the inner angle of your elbow should slightly increase as the punch travels forward. Retract and then repeat using your lead hand for the second body shot. Rotate around the waist, shift your rear shoulder forward, pivot on the ball of the rear foot, and extend your rear arm to throw the cross. Lift and lock your lead elbow at 90 degrees and rotate around the waist to throw the lead hook.

COMBINATION 52
Jab, slip, uppercut, hook, cross
Retract the jab and slip adjacent to your rear hand, taking your head off the center line. Throw the rear uppercut followed by the lead hook and cross.

COMBINATION 53
Jab, cross, slip step across yourself with lead foot, counter hook
To slip step across yourself, you have to make sure that the lead foot crosses your center line. Shift your lead shoulder forward as you slip to the side adjacent to your rear knee and then step your lead foot across your center line. Pivot on the ball of your lead foot to reset your feet. Lift and lock your lead elbow at 90 degrees as you rotate around the waist to throw the counter hook.

COMBINATION 54
Jab, cross, hook, shuffle to lateral side of target, hook
After retracting the first hook, shuffle your feet to the side adjacent to your rear foot to position yourself on the lateral side of your target. Throw a second hook.

TRAINING REGIMENS

Anytime you embark on a fitness journey with a new training regimen, it's very important to start with a gradual approach to ensure longevity and realize long-term success. Whether you are a beginner or are an experienced fitness enthusiast looking to add something different to your workout, be patient and consistent to allow yourself time to gradually increase and maintain performance. This chapter includes a sample weekly training regimen for beginner, intermediate, and experienced fitness enthusiasts to help you shape out your training week. For freestyle shadowboxing and freestyle heavy bag rounds, you can choose from the combinations listed in Chapter 7 or create your own.

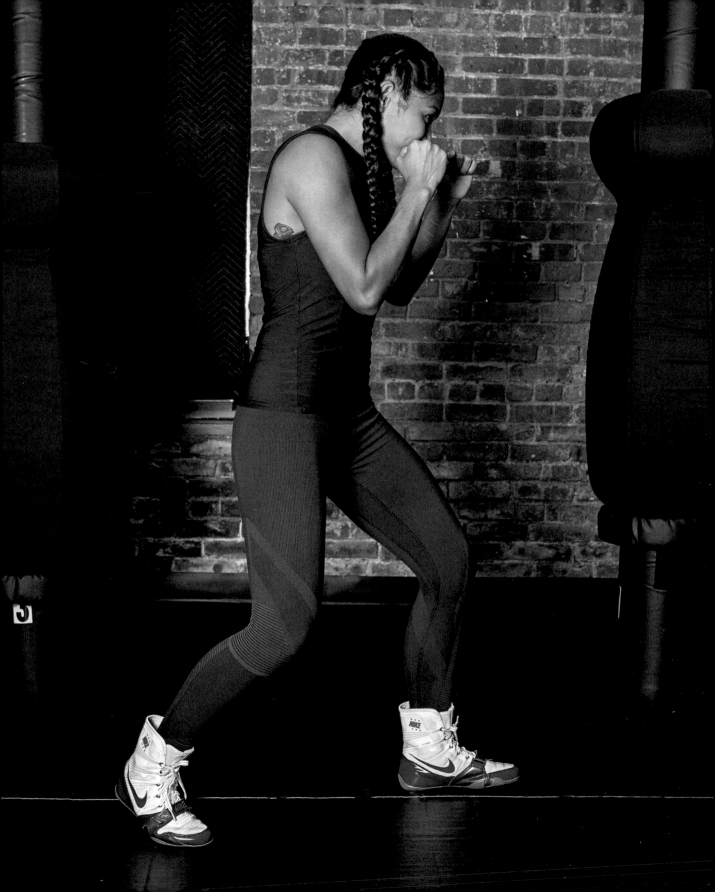

BEGINNER SAMPLE I

DAY 1

Road work and warm-up: 1.5-mile run.

Shadowboxing: Do 3 freestyle shadowboxing rounds. Set a boxing timer to a 3-minute round with a 1-minute rest period in between rounds.

Heavy bag: Do 4 freestyle rounds on the heavy bag. Set a boxing timer to a 3-minute round with a 1-minute rest period in between rounds.

Cool-down: Jump rope for 6 minutes.

DAY 2

Rest and recover.

DAY 3

Road work and warm-up: 1.5-mile run.

Shadowboxing: Do 3 freestyle shadowboxing rounds. Set a boxing timer to a 2-minute round with a 1-minute rest period in between rounds.

Heavy bag: Do 3 freestyle rounds on the heavy bag. Set a boxing timer to a 2-minute round with a 1-minute rest period in between rounds.

Push-Ups (page 58): 5 sets of 10 repetitions

Pull-Ups (page 59): 5 sets of 10 repetitions

Dips (page 60): 5 sets of 10 repetitions

DAY 4

Rest and recover.

DAY 5

Warm-up: Jump rope for 8 minutes.

Pendulum steps (pages 27–30) and Cutting off the Ring (page 33): Practice for 3 rounds. Set a boxing timer to a 3-minute round with a 1-minute rest period in between rounds.

Shadowboxing: Shadowbox for 6 rounds incorporating specific defense drills. Set a boxing timer to a 3-minute round with a 1-minute rest period in between rounds. Review drills in Chapter 3.

- Rounds 1 and 4: Incorporate slipping punches (slip/dip/pull back/pivot/weave) and catch and throw.
- Rounds 2 and 5: Incorporate parrying, countering, and level changing.
- Rounds 3 and 6: Incorporate retreat and circle and retreat and counter.

DAY 6

Rest and recover.

DAY 7

Rest and recover.

BEGINNER SAMPLE II

DAY 1

Road work and warm-up: 1.5-mile run.

Shadowboxing: Do 3 freestyle shadowboxing rounds. Set a boxing timer to a 3-minute round with a 1-minute rest period in between rounds.

Heavy bag: Do 4 freestyle rounds on the heavy bag. Set a boxing timer to a 3-minute round with a 1-minute rest period in between rounds.

Cool-down: Jump rope for 6 minutes.

DAY 2

Rest and recover.

DAY 3

Warm-up: Light jog on treadmill for 1 mile.

Treadmill Sprints (page 63): Do 10 repetitions; sprint 10 seconds; rest 20 seconds (5 minutes).

Heavy Bag Drill (page 64): Do 10 rounds; work 1 minute; rest 10 seconds (12 minutes).

Push-Ups (page 58): 5 sets of 10 repetitions

Pull-Ups (page 59): 5 sets of 10 repetitions

Dips (page 60): 5 sets of 10 repetitions

DAY 4

Rest and recover.

DAY 5

Warm-up: Jump rope for 8 minutes.

Pendulum steps (pages 27–30) and Cutting off the Ring (page 33): Practice for 3 rounds. Set a boxing timer to a 3-minute round with a 1-minute rest period in between rounds.

Shadowboxing: Shadowbox for 6 rounds incorporating specific defense drills. Set a boxing timer to a 3-minute round with a 1-minute rest period in between rounds. Review drills in Chapter 3.

- Rounds 1 and 4: Incorporate slipping punches (slip/dip/pull back/pivot/weave) and catch and throw.

- Rounds 2 and 5: Incorporate parrying, countering, and level changing.

- Rounds 3 and 6: Incorporate retreat and circle and retreat and counter.

DAY 6

Rest and recover.

DAY 7

Rest and recover.

BEGINNER SAMPLE III

DAY 1

Road work and warm-up: 1.5-mile run.

Shadowboxing: Do 3 freestyle shadowboxing rounds with 2-pound dumbbells. Set a boxing timer to a 3-minute round with a 1-minute rest period in between rounds.

Shadowboxing: Shadowbox for 5 rounds incorporating specific footwork drills. Set a boxing timer to a 3-minute round with a 1-minute rest period in between rounds.

- Round 1: Uppercuts moving forward and backward (pages 21–22)

- Round 2: Jab and Cross Moving Side to Side (page 23)

- Round 3: Jab Moving Forward and Backward (page 24) and Jab and Cross Moving Side to Side (page 23)

- Round 4: Jab and Rear Uppercut with Rear Step Off (page 25) and Cross and Lead Hook with Lead Step Off (page 26)

- Round 5: Pendulum steps (pages 27–30)

Calisthenic Round:

- Kick-Back Burpee to Plank Push-Up (page 69), 1 minute

- Jump Squat (page 62), 1 minute

- Mountain Climber Burpee (page 70), 1 minute

Core Work: 4 sets

- Crunch of choice (pages 74–75), 1 minute

- 360-Degree Abs (page 76): Hold each position for 30 seconds before rotating into next position, 2 minutes

DAY 2

Rest and recover.

DAY 3

Warm-up: Light jog on treadmill for 1 mile.

Treadmill Sprints (page 63): Do 10 repetitions; sprint 10 seconds; rest 20 seconds (5 minutes).

Heavy Bag Drill (page 64): Do 10 rounds; work 1 minute; rest 10 seconds (12 minutes).

Push-Ups (page 58): 5 sets of 10 repetitions

Pull-Ups (page 59): 5 sets of 10 repetitions

Dips (page 60): 5 sets of 10 repetitions

DAY 4

Rest and recover.

DAY 5

Warm-up: Jump rope for 8 minutes.

Pendulum steps (pages 27–30) and Cutting off the Ring (page 33): Practice for 3 rounds. Set a boxing timer to a 3-minute round with a 1-minute rest period in between rounds.

Shadowboxing: Shadowbox for 6 rounds incorporating specific defense drills. Set a boxing timer to a 3-minute round with a 1-minute rest period in between rounds. Review drills in Chapter 3.

- Rounds 1 and 4: Incorporate slipping punches (slip/dip/pull back/pivot/weave) and catch and throw.

- Rounds 2 and 5: Incorporate parrying, countering, and level changing.

- Rounds 3 and 6: Incorporate retreat and circle and retreat and counter.

DAY 6

Rest and recover.

DAY 7

Rest and recover.

INTERMEDIATE SAMPLE I

DAY 1

Road work and warm-up: 2-mile run.

Shadowboxing: Do 3 freestyle shadowboxing rounds. Set a boxing timer to a 3-minute round with a 1-minute rest period in between rounds.

Heavy bag: Do 6 freestyle rounds on the heavy bag. Set a boxing timer to a 3-minute round with a 1-minute rest period in between rounds.

Cool-down: Jump rope for 6 to 8 minutes.

DAY 2

Rest and recover.

DAY 3

Road work and warm-up: 2-mile run.

Shadowboxing: Do 4 freestyle shadowboxing rounds. Set a boxing timer to a 2-minute round with a 1-minute rest period in between rounds.

Heavy bag: Do 4 freestyle rounds on the heavy bag. Set a boxing timer to a 2-minute round with a 1-minute rest period in between rounds.

Push-Ups (page 58): 5 sets of 10 repetitions

Pull-Ups (page 59): 5 sets of 10 repetitions

Dips (page 60): 5 sets of 10 repetitions

DAY 4

Circuit I (page 98).

DAY 5

Rest and recover.

DAY 6

Warm-up: Jump rope for 8 minutes.

Pendulum steps (pages 27–30) and Cutting off the Ring (page 33): Practice for 3 rounds. Set a boxing timer to a 3-minute round with a 1-minute rest period in between rounds.

Shadowboxing: Shadowbox for 6 rounds incorporating specific defense drills. Set a boxing timer to a 3-minute round with a 1-minute rest period in between rounds. Review drills in Chapter 3.

- Rounds 1 and 4: Incorporate slipping punches (slip/dip/pull back/pivot/weave) and catch and throw.

- Rounds 2 and 5: Incorporate parrying, countering, and level changing.

- Rounds 3 and 6: Incorporate retreat and circle and retreat and counter.

DAY 7

Rest and recover.

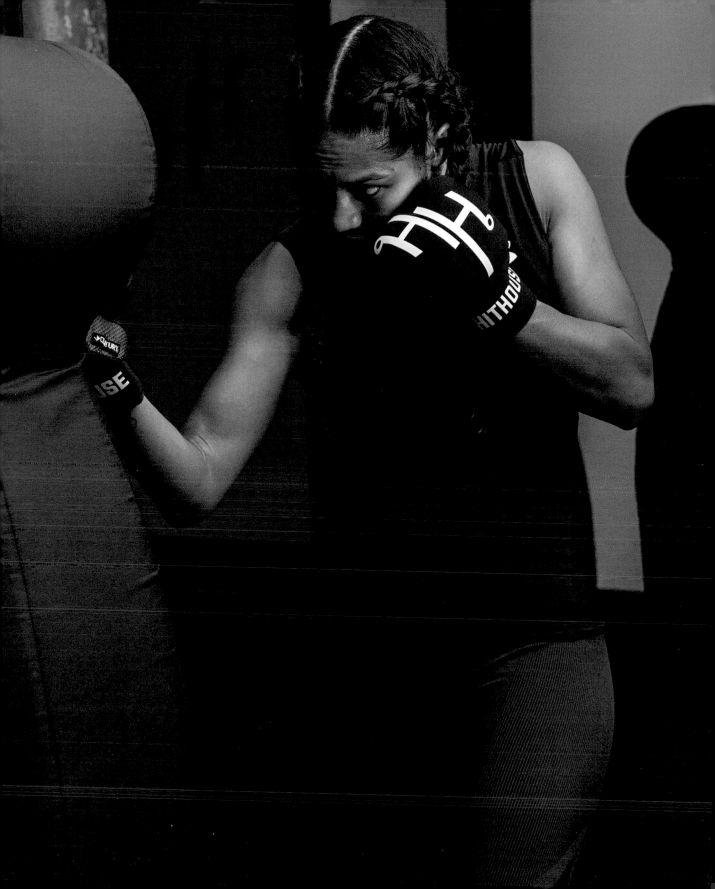

INTERMEDIATE SAMPLE II

DAY 1

Road work and warm-up: 2-mile run.

Shadowboxing: Do 3 freestyle shadowboxing rounds. Set a boxing timer to a 3-minute round with a 1-minute rest period in between rounds.

Heavy bag: Do 6 freestyle rounds on the heavy bag. Set a boxing timer to a 3-minute round with a 1-minute rest period in between rounds.

Cool-down: Jump rope for 6 to 8 minutes.

DAY 2

Rest and recover.

DAY 3

Warm-up: Light jog on treadmill for 1.5 miles.

Treadmill Sprints (page 63): Do 10 repetitions; sprint 20 seconds; rest 10 seconds (5 minutes).

Heavy Bag Drill (page 64): Do 10 rounds; work 1 minute; rest 10 seconds (12 minutes).

Push-Ups (page 58): 5 sets of 10 repetitions

Pull-Ups (page 59): 5 sets of 10 repetitions

Dips (page 60): 5 sets of 10 repetitions

DAY 4

Circuit I (page 98).

DAY 5

Rest and recover.

DAY 6

Warm-up: Jump rope for 8 minutes.

Pendulum steps (pages 27–30) and Cutting off the Ring (page 33): Practice for 3 rounds. Set a boxing timer to a 3-minute round with a 1-minute rest period in between rounds.

Shadowboxing: Shadowbox for 6 rounds incorporating specific defense drills. Set a boxing timer to a 3-minute round with a 1-minute rest period in between rounds. Review drills in Chapter 3.

- Rounds 1 and 4: Incorporate slipping punches (slip/dip/pull back/pivot/weave) and catch and throw.

- Rounds 2 and 5: Incorporate parrying, countering, and level changing.

- Rounds 3 and 6: Incorporate retreat and circle and retreat and counter.

DAY 7

Rest and recover.

INTERMEDIATE SAMPLE III

DAY 1

Road work and warm-up: 2-mile run.

Shadowboxing: Do 3 freestyle shadowboxing rounds. Set a boxing timer to a 3-minute round with a 1-minute rest period in between rounds.

Heavy bag: Do 6 freestyle rounds on the heavy bag. Set a boxing timer to a 3-minute round with a 1-minute rest period in between rounds.

Cool-down: Jump rope for 6 to 8 minutes.

DAY 2

Rest and recover.

DAY 3

Warm-up: Light jog on treadmill for 1.5 miles.

Treadmill Sprints (page 63): Do 10 repetitions; sprint 20 seconds; rest 10 seconds (5 minutes).

Heavy Bag Drill (page 64): Do 10 rounds; work 1 minute; rest 10 seconds (12 minutes).

Push-Ups (page 58): 5 sets of 10 repetitions

Pull-Ups (page 59): 5 sets of 10 repetitions

Dips (page 60): 5 sets of 10 repetitions

DAY 4

Circuit I (page 98).

DAY 5

Rest and recover.

DAY 6

Warm-up: Jump rope for 8 minutes.

Pendulum steps (pages 27–30) and Cutting off the Ring (page 33): Practice for 3 rounds. Set a boxing timer to a 3-minute round with a 1-minute rest period in between rounds.

Shadowboxing: Shadowbox for 6 rounds incorporating specific defense drills. Set a boxing timer to a 3-minute round with a 1-minute rest period in between rounds. Review drills in Chapter 3.

- Rounds 1 and 4: Incorporate slipping punches (slip/dip/pull back/pivot/weave) and catch and throw.
- Rounds 2 and 5: Incorporate parrying, countering, and level changing.
- Rounds 3 and 6: Incorporate retreat and circle and retreat and counter.

DAY 7

Road work and warm-up: 1.5-mile run.

Shadowboxing: Do 3 freestyle shadowboxing rounds with 2-pound dumbbells. Set a boxing timer to a 3-minute round with a 1-minute rest period in between rounds.

Shadowboxing: Shadowbox for 5 rounds incorporating specific footwork drills. Set a boxing timer to a 3-minute round with a 1-minute rest period in between rounds.

- Round 1: Uppercuts moving forward and backward (pages 21–22).
- Round 2: Jab and Cross Moving Side to Side (page 23).
- Round 3: Jab Moving Forward and Backward (page 24) and Jab and Cross Moving Side to Side (page 23)
- Round 4: Jab and Rear Uppercut with Rear Step Off (page 25) and Cross and Lead Hook with Lead Step Off (page 26)
- Round 5: Pendulum steps (pages 27–30)

Calisthenic Round:
- Kick-Back Burpee to Plank Push-Up (page 69), 1 minute
- Jump Squat (page 62), 1 minute
- Mountain Climber Burpee (page 70), 1 minute

Core Work: 4 sets
- Crunch of choice (pages 74–75), 1 minute
- 360-Degree Abs (page 76): Hold each position for 30 seconds before rotating into next position, 2 minutes

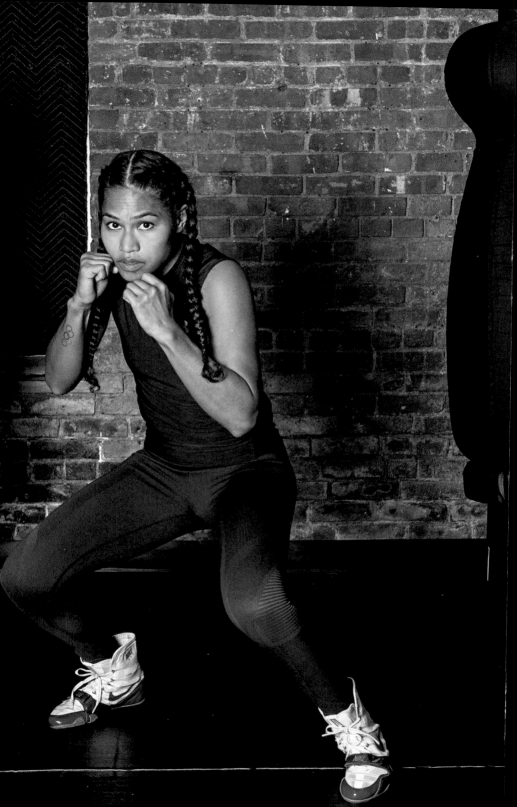

EXPERIENCED SAMPLE I

DAY 1

Road work and warm-up: 2-mile run.

Shadowboxing: Do 3 freestyle shadowboxing rounds. Set a boxing timer to a 3-minute round with a 1-minute rest period in between rounds.

Heavy bag: Do 6 freestyle rounds on the heavy bag. Set a boxing timer to a 3-minute round with a 1-minute rest period in between rounds.

Cool-down: Jump rope for 6 to 8 minutes.

DAY 2

Circuit I (page 98).

DAY 3

Road work and warm-up: 2-mile run.

Shadowboxing: Do 4 freestyle shadowboxing rounds. Set a boxing timer to a 2-minute round with a 1-minute rest period in between rounds.

Heavy bag: Do 4 freestyle rounds on the heavy bag. Set a boxing timer to a 2-minute round with a 1-minute rest period in between rounds.

Push-Ups (page 58): 5 sets of 10 repetitions

Pull-Ups (page 59): 5 sets of 10 repetitions

Dips (page 60): 5 sets of 10 repetitions

DAY 4

Circuit II (page 100).

DAY 5

Warm-up: Jump rope for 8 minutes.

Pendulum steps (pages 27–30) and Cutting off the Ring (page 33): Practice for 3 rounds. Set a boxing timer to a 3-minute round with a 1-minute rest period in between rounds.

Shadowboxing: Shadowbox for 6 rounds incorporating specific defense drills. Set a boxing timer to a 3-minute round with a 1-minute rest period in between rounds. Review drills in Chapter 3.

- Rounds 1 and 4: Incorporate slipping punches (slip/dip/pull back/pivot/weave) and catch and throw.

- Rounds 2 and 5: Incorporate parrying, countering, and level changing.

- Rounds 3 and 6: Incorporate retreat and circle and retreat and counter.

DAY 6

Warm-up: Jump rope for 8 minutes.

Endurance: Circuit III (page 101).

DAY 7

Rest and recover.

EXPERIENCED SAMPLE II

DAY 1

Road work and warm-up: 2-mile run.

Shadowboxing: Do 3 freestyle shadowboxing rounds. Set a boxing timer to a 3-minute round with a 1-minute rest period in between rounds.

Heavy bag: Do 6 freestyle rounds on the heavy bag. Set a boxing timer to a 3-minute round with a 1-minute rest period in between rounds.

Cool-down: Jump rope for 6 to 8 minutes.

DAY 2

Circuit I (page 98).

DAY 3

Warm-up: Light jog on treadmill for 1.5 miles.

Treadmill Sprints (page 63): Do 10 repetitions; sprint 30 seconds; rest 30 seconds (10 minutes).

Heavy Bag Drill (page 64): Do 10 rounds; work 1 minute; rest 10 seconds (12 minutes).

Push-Ups (page 58): 5 sets of 10 repetitions

Pull-Ups (page 59): 5 sets of 10 repetitions

Dips (page 60): 5 sets of 10 repetitions

DAY 4

Circuit II (page 100).

DAY 5

Warm-up: Jump rope for 8 minutes.

Pendulum steps (pages 27–30) and Cutting off the Ring (page 33): Practice for 3 rounds. Set a boxing timer to a 3-minute round with a 1-minute rest period in between rounds.

Shadowboxing: Do 6 rounds incorporating specific defense drills. Set a boxing timer to a 3-minute round with a 1-minute rest period in between rounds. Review drills in Chapter 3.

- Rounds 1 and 4: Incorporate slipping punches (slip/dip/pull back/pivot/weave) and catch and throw.

- Rounds 2 and 5: Incorporate parrying, countering, and level changing.

- Rounds 3 and 6: Incorporate retreat and circle and retreat and counter.

DAY 6

Warm-up: Jump rope for 8 minutes.

Endurance: Circuit III (page 101).

DAY 7

Rest and recover.

EXPERIENCED SAMPLE III

DAY 1

Road work and warm-up: 2-mile run.

Shadowboxing: Do 3 freestyle shadowboxing rounds. Set a boxing timer to a 3-minute round with a 1-minute rest period in between rounds.

Heavy bag: Do 4 freestyle rounds on the heavy bag. Set a boxing timer to a 3-minute round with a 1-minute rest period in between rounds.

Shadowboxing: Shadowbox for 5 rounds incorporating specific footwork drills. Set a boxing timer to a 3-minute round with a 1-minute rest period in between rounds.

- Round 1: Uppercuts moving forward and backward (pages 21–22)
- Round 2: Jab and Cross Moving Side to Side (page 23).
- Round 3: Jab Moving Forward and Backward (page 24) and Jab and Cross Moving Side to Side (page 23).
- Round 4: Jab and Rear Uppercut with Rear Step Off (page 25) and Cross and Lead Hook with Lead Step Off (page 26)
- Round 5: Pendulum steps (pages 27–30)

Calisthenic Round:

- Kick-Back Burpee to Plank Push-Up (page 69), 1 minute
- Jump Squat (page 62), 1 minute
- Mountain Climber Burpee (page 70), 1 minute

Core Work: 4 sets

- Crunch of choice (pages 74–75), 1 minute
- 360-Degree Abs (page 76): Hold each position for 30 seconds before rotating into next position, 2 minutes

DAY 2

Circuit I (page 98).

DAY 3

Warm-up: Light jog on treadmill for 1.5 miles.

Treadmill Sprints (page 63): Do 10 repetitions; sprint 30 seconds; rest 30 seconds (10 minutes).

Heavy Bag Drill (page 64): Do 10 rounds; work 1 minute; rest 10 seconds (12 minutes).

Push-Ups (page 58): 5 sets of 10 repetitions

Pull-Ups (page 59): 5 sets of 10 repetitions

Dips (page 60): 5 sets of 10 repetitions

DAY 4

Circuit II (page 100).

DAY 5

Warm-up: Jump rope for 8 minutes.

Pendulum steps (pages 27–30) and Cutting off the Ring (page 33): Practice for 3 rounds. Set a boxing timer to a 3-minute round with a 1-minute rest period in between rounds.

Shadowboxing: Shadowbox for 6 rounds incorporating specific defense drills. Set a boxing timer to a 3-minute round with a 1-minute rest period in between rounds. Review drills in Chapter 3.

- Rounds 1 and 4: Incorporate slipping punches (slip/dip/pull back/pivot/weave) and catch and throw.
- Rounds 2 and 5: Incorporate parrying, countering, and level changing.
- Rounds 3 and 6: Incorporate retreat and circle and retreat and counter.

DAY 6

Warm-up: Jump rope for 8 minutes.

Endurance: Circuit III (page 101).

DAY 7

Rest and recover.

INDEX

ACKNOWLEDGMENTS

First and foremost, thank you to the publishing team at Ulysses, especially Bridget Thoreson and Claire Sielaff, whose guidance throughout this project helped shape the concept of this book to make it the best it can be.

I am grateful to my dedicated team; my photographer Joshua Brandenburg, my teammates Raquel Harris, Bridget Grace, and Henry Lee, whose time, effort, and feedback this project could not be completed without.

Finally, thank you to my son, Adam, and to my dearest friend, Faidat Olayide Fahm, for your ever encouraging support.

ABOUT THE AUTHOR

Jennifer Dugwen Chieng is a professional athlete and former Olympic boxer who represented the Federated States of Micronesia (FSM) in the 2016 Rio Olympics. In 2015, she became the first female athlete and boxer from the FSM to win gold at the Pacific Games, the premier multi-sport event in the Oceania region incepted in 1963.

She transitioned from Olympic boxing to mixed martial arts (MMA) in October 2016 and made her professional MMA debut on October 13, 2018, under Bellator MMA, winning her professional debut. She currently resides in Brooklyn, New York.

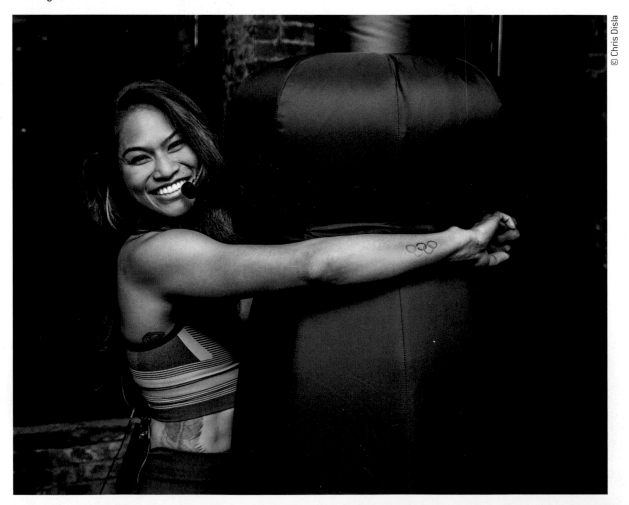

© Chris Disla